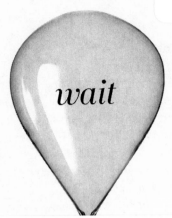

wait

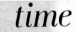

time

Life Writing Series

In the Life Writing Series, Wilfrid Laurier University Press publishes life writing and new life-writing criticism and theory in order to promote autobiographical accounts, diaries, letters, memoirs and testimonials written and/or told by women and men whose political, literary, or philosophical purposes are central to their lives. The Series features accounts written in English, or translated into English from French or the languages of the First Nations, or any of the languages of immigration to Canada.

The audience for the series includes scholars, youth, and avid general readers both in Canada and abroad. The Series hopes to continue its work as a leading publisher of life writing of all kinds, as an imprint that aims for scholarly excellence and representing lived experience as tools for both historical and autobiographical research.

We publish original life writing which represents the widest range of experiences of lives lived with integrity. Life Writing also publishes original theoretical investigations about life writing, as long as they are not limited to one author or text.

Series Editor
Marlene Kadar
Humanities, York University

Manuscripts to be sent to
Lisa Quinn, Acquisitions Editor
Wilfrid Laurier University Press
75 University Avenue West
Waterloo, Ontario N2L 3C5, Canada

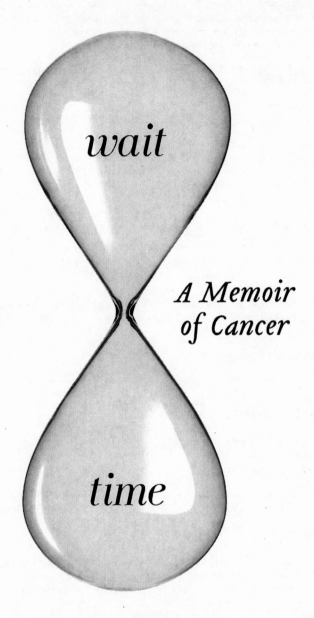

wait

A Memoir of Cancer

time

Kenneth Sherman

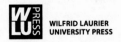

WILFRID LAURIER UNIVERSITY PRESS

Wilfrid Laurier University Press acknowledges the support of the Canada Council for the Arts for our publishing program. We acknowledge the financial support of the Government of Canada through the Canada Book Fund for our publishing activities. This work was supported by the Research Support Fund.

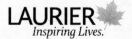 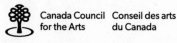

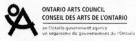

Library and Archives Canada Cataloguing in Publication

Sherman, Kenneth, 1950–, author
    Wait time / Kenneth Sherman.

(Life writing)
Issued in print and electronic formats.

ISBN 978-1-77112-188-0 (paperback).—ISBN 978-1-77112-189-7 (pdf).—
ISBN 978-1-77112-190-3 (epub)

    1. Sherman, Kenneth, 1950– —Health. 2. Cancer—Patients—Canada—Biography.
3. Poets, Canadian (English)—20th century—Biography. I. Title. II. Series: Life writing
series

PS8587.H3863Z53 2016   C811'.54   C2015-905583-0
                                                                    C2015-905584-9

Cover design by Sandra Friesen. Cover image by Ziviani, *hourglass*, iStock photo.
Text design by Mike Bechthold.

This book is printed on FSC® certified paper and is certified Ecologo. It contains post-consumer fibre, is processed chlorine free, and is manufactured using biogas energy.

Printed in Canada

Every reasonable effort has been made to acquire permission for copyright material used in this text, and to acknowledge all such indebtedness accurately. Any errors and omissions called to the publisher's attention will be corrected in future printings.

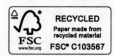

Sickness sensitizes man for observation, like a photographic plate.
>—Edmond and Jules de Goncourt
>(*Journals*, 1865)

There is, let us confess it (and illness is the great confessional), a childish outspokenness in illness; things are said, truths blurted out, which the cautious respectability of health conceals.
>—Virginia Woolf ("On Being Ill," 1926)

The patient has to start by treating his illness not as a disaster, an occasion for depression or panic, but as a narrative, a story.
>—Anatole Broyard (*Intoxicated by My Illness*, 1992)

Contents

Foreword

Kenneth Sherman is a writer. But with this publication he is also a subject, a patient. As the subject, he patiently writes from the point of view of timekeeper—the person who measures time in order to call "time's up" should the time limits be exceeded. He keeps time as he waits to find out how ill he is, which treatments he must endure, and ultimately how long he might have to live: What is the rate of OS (overall survival) in his case? What are the time limits?

Sherman's endurance is measured by his method of note-taking. The book is metred by a collection of dated entries that begins with his first medical appointment and ends with a brief meditation on time and how it means differently to those whose time has come to enter the world of the healthy.

Waiting to hear from physicians about the state of one's health is both a blessing and a trial by fire. Most of the time we are told not to worry while we wait, which every good, mature human being will try to accomplish; and most of the time the news is good, or neutral, and requires no further expenditure of emotion or pain or waiting.

But sometimes the news is not good. Sometimes it is a diagnosis of cancer, the word that was once only whispered, not even spoken out loud.

Sherman does suffer getting the bad news (finally) that he has kidney cancer and that the cancer has spread to a bone, a single rib. Adjusting to such news is difficult for him, as it would be for anyone; but because Sherman is both a patient and a scholar, he is able to write, with expression and nuance, about his experience, and about the disease and the feelings that accompany it, and about numerous other wise patients who became narrators of illness. He is particularly aware of philosophers whose own diagnoses of cancer provided the fodder for their first-person narrations.

Sherman experiences a sea change of identity as soon as he learns he is a sick man. Before that moment, on March 18, 2010, he is waiting for a diagnosis; after that moment he is waiting for health, ideally to be disease-free—which is not always possible when cells exchange normalcy for malignancy rapidly and energetically. The institution of Medicine and those who agree to uphold it and apply it are in the arduous position of keeping up with these cells as best they can without always being able to see them, measure them, target them, halt them, kill them. As Sherman says elsewhere, these cells are more vigorous and intelligent than their vanquished brother and sister cells. He refers to Siddhartha Mukherjee, the highly regarded author of *The Emperor of All Maladies: A Biography of Cancer*, who insists that cancer is "a parallel species ... more adapted to survival than we are" (63–64).

A change of another sort occurs on March 18, 2010, too. Sherman that day becomes a patient with a potentially death-dealing illness and also a writer who uses his illness to fuel a creative act. Luckily for other patients and readers, Sherman embarks on an extemporization. "Once the doctor tells you you are ill, you begin to eke out your existence as a patient. Your life becomes an improvisation around the theme of illness" (46). For me, that improvisation is the only saving grace in what other narrators have called their "cancer journey"— a ubiquitous and tedious phrase used to give the personal experience of a cancer a metre, a continuum respecting its development through stages and types. To improvise is to write around the event, an event that does not often have a foreseeable end, and if it is deemed a happy ending by good readers of this book, it is not as comforting as happy endings are meant to be. The ending, of course, is of necessity made up. There is a lull: we have made progress; things are much better; the side effects are nothing when compared to the disease. And yet most patients I know live in the middle of this lull where arguably the main concern is the return—the return of the same cancer or of another cancer—or the appearance of a different "transformed" disease or a new cancer induced by the treatment.

Sherman counters Susan Sontag's warnings about thinking in metaphors—Sontag says that as a cancer patient she swore off metaphors. But Sherman cannot do this. "The truth is," he writes, "once you hear the news of your illness, the metaphoric thinking begins. It rarely lets up" (62). And, *pace* Sontag, he thinks, "the terror of my imaginings keeps me phoning for earlier appointments, quicker results" (64). He figures out that the wait time for surgery at the prestigious Princess Margaret Hospital, in Toronto, is eighty-five days and that at Woodstock General, a short distance away, it is only twenty-three days. His research inspires him to plead with doctors and their assistants for an earlier date, in order that he wait less. While he waits, of course, his illness does not stand still: "I know full well that the cancer could be spreading to other bones and organs" (69). Waiting is nothing short of dangerous.

And yet waiting for the cancer to return is part and parcel of life after diagnosis and after treatments that have their own risks. They kill good cells as well as malignant cells, so the ultimate wait time is for the return of cancer in one form or another. It doesn't always return, but the spectre hangs over patients. In spite of this ultimate irony, Sherman knows he will forget about his illness. He will soon become a member of the land of the well, where different rules and provisos prevail and where illusions about mortality and wellness dominate. On the last page of the book, he writes: "With time, our scars fade. Memory fades, too. My fear is that as the months and years pass I will become complacent and careless with Time. I will see Time as those who are blessed with health see it: an unending horizon.... I will forget what I learned when I looked back from the edge of life" (126).

There is another irony in the orbit of "wait time." Waiting carries with it some hope, because every visit to a cancer hospital brings both relief and sorrow and often in the same breath, the same moment, the same action. "No matter what the actual result, it hurts to wait, and it hurts not to wait because waiting means you are alive and not waiting means you don't have to wait anymore" (Kadar, October 7, 2015, oncologist's waiting room). What else does it mean?

At one point in his diagnosis, Sherman tries to confront the imaginary pain he feels in his ribs. He knows it is imaginary because until he is told the rib is involved he had had no pain there whatsoever. This gives rise to the thought "I wonder how I will manage to cope with the physical disease if I can't get my mind back in order" (27). By the end of the memoir, Sherman does have his mind back in order, he does "manage to cope with the physical disease," and the story comes to a happyish ending. I say "-ish" only because the cancer patient waits interminably for a treated cancer to return, or for the treatment itself to generate yet another illness, while also taking solace in the waiting: I am alive, he says, I am living, I belong again to the world of the well, where another set of rules applies, but I am also forever looking "back from the edge."

A profoundly sensitive and honest ending to the story.

—Marlene Kadar,
12 October 2015

Preface

This book began as a notebook that I kept when I was diagnosed with renal-cell carcinoma (kidney cancer) in the spring of 2010. Two years before, I had written an essay on the subject of illness and literature titled "The Angel of Disease," which appeared first in the journal *Ars Medica* and later in my collection *What the Furies Bring*. As I was to discover, writing about illness from the vantage point of health is markedly different from writing about it as a cancer patient.

My reading on the subject in no way prepared me for the emotional upheaval I was to endure once I was diagnosed. The experience did, however, shed a clearer light on the intent of those authors who had dealt first-hand with the subject of illness. I was now in their circle and could understand their anxieties; I could appreciate their grasping for the least shred of hope. In the midst of my turmoil, their words took on a vital urgency.

Some time after my operation, I began expanding the notes I had kept and saw the possibility of a book. Keeping a notebook while I attended doctors' appointments and underwent tests helped preserve my sanity. And the writing of my book proved to be therapeutic: like any patient, I had intense emotions as well as strong opinions that I longed to express regarding my cancer experience.

When I sent my manuscript out in search of a publisher I had no idea how reluctant editors would be to consider a book about illness. In 1978, Susan Sontag called cancer a "scandalous subject." It still is. It is far more scandalous than sex or dirty politics. I was to discover that illness, along with death, is our society's forbidden subject. At the root of our repugnance is fear, and it is fear that accounts for our inability to incorporate death into our lives as a meaningful experience. Since serious illness is often viewed as the antechamber to death, it too is a subject that is denied at all costs.

Why revisit wounds? When I came to revise my book, I found it a painful experience, reliving the trauma of the past, going over events and observations I'd buried. What kept me going was the belief that others would benefit from hearing my tale. When I was a traveller in the land of cancer, my greatest consolation came from the support and love of my immediate family and friends. But I was likewise steadied by the testimonies and observations of those writers who had travelled the wild terrain before me and had composed their reports. Some were written as these authors lay dying.

Their courage, honesty, and insights were a tremendous help to me in my time of need and if this book can be of similar service to the recently diagnosed, then the work will have been worthwhile.

—Kenneth Sherman,
Toronto 2015

Part One

Tuesday, March 16

I can hear myself breathe.

I can hear the examination paper crinkle under my back as my general practitioner, Dr. Sidney Nusinowitz, presses down repeatedly on my abdomen. His friendly banter stops. I know something is not right even before Sid says in a low voice: "I can feel your spleen." He follows with an aside, almost as if he were speaking to himself: "I shouldn't be able to feel your spleen." His eyes—usually bright and playful—narrow with concern behind his dark-framed glasses. He presses again and again along my lower abdomen, then in one swift motion sits down on his swivel stool and picks up the phone. He says—in a low voice as he dials—that he is booking me an ultrasound appointment, but I am too frightened to ask what he suspects might be the problem. He reports that there is an opening at the ultrasound clinic the next day, and I tell him that I am scheduled to administer a test at the college where I am teaching. Of course, I ought to take the appointment and ask someone to substitute for me, if only to limit the wait time and the worry I will have to endure. But duty is in play—or fear of knowing—and I ask Sid if it is all right to postpone the ultrasound a few days. He nods and books me an appointment for later in the week.

There is tension in the tiny room as Sid sits and types into his computer, making notes on my file. I study his pursed lips, his furrowed brow, his concentrated gaze at the computer screen. I study his muteness. Psychologists consider the moment of diagnosis for a deadly disease to be a traumatic event; the trauma starts early and builds as you pick up body signals and interpret silences.

Without looking up, Sid requests a urine sample. I walk numbly down the hall to the washroom, and then return with the warm container into which Sid drops a test strip and reports that my urine is normal. When I finally do work up the nerve to ask what he thinks the problem is, he tells me he doesn't know, but he's sure it is "nothing serious." Do I believe him? I trust him as a doctor, but I do not believe him. There is an ever-so-slight note of apprehension in his voice, and I am too distressed to press him, to find out what list of possibilities he is running through in his mind. In any event, what would I gain by hearing his conjectures? There is nothing to do, really, but wait to have the ultrasound and wait for the results.

Waiting, as I am about to discover, is what being a patient is mostly about.

8

What do you do after leaving a doctor's office when there has been an unsettling and unresolved discovery?

Drive home, crawl into bed, and pull the comforter over your face?

Marie, my wife, has given me a list of grocery items to pick up after my doctor's appointment. I drive a short distance to the Metro supermarket, and as I take hold of the rattling buggy I call home on my cellphone. I tell Marie—trying to sound my usual self but likely failing—that the appointment has not gone well. When she—concerned and sympathetic—suggests that I drive home, I respond that I will do the shopping first.

"Are you sure?" she asks.

I am not sure, but it seems best to try and preserve normalcy. As I put the phone back into my pocket and grab hold of the buggy, I wonder if my actions are a sign of good mental health—the ability to maintain routine in the face of adversity—or a means of denial. I pull a folded piece of note-paper from my back pocket. It is from one of those notepads that charities send out. Marie's name and mine are blazoned on the top in bold blue script and underneath, in Marie's elegant cursive, is the list:

Greek low-fat yogourt
organic strawberries
Bob's steel-cut oats
unsalted almonds
green tea

Hardly a list for a couple courting ill health.

In the dairy aisle I pick up a tub of yogourt and then, as I make my way to the fruits and vegetables, I halt.

I am three months shy of sixty; I am at an age where things, medically speaking, might start going awry, though they aren't supposed to happen to me.

I run five kilometres three days a week.

I do yoga.

I have no symptoms.

Where I happen to be shopping is a supermarket in the Lawrence Plaza, a place I often walked as a boy in the mid-1950s. I have no hard evidence that I am near death or even ill, yet my life at this moment seems poignantly bracketed by this L-shaped plaza of unremarkable stores. The building housing the supermarket where I am standing was once Morgan's, a department store. My mother took me there to buy winter mittens and a wool hat to protect me from the cold. It's no coincidence that I'm recalling a time when I was protected from the elements, since I'm feeling vulnerable, defenceless. The Morgan's store is long gone, as is Jack's Restaurant across the parking lot. On nights when my father worked late, my mother would take my younger sister and me to Jack's. I would order a butterscotch sundae for dessert; it came topped with whipped cream and a maraschino cherry. I had my first hair-cut at the Lawrence Plaza barbershop. My barber's name was

Vince: he wore a greased Elvis Presley ducktail and had a deep scar running down from the corner of his mouth. I first heard Elvis's "Heartbreak Hotel" on the radio in Vince's shop, Vince softly echoing the words in his Sicilian accent; I was unaware at the time that Elvis's hotel was a place where, sooner or later, we all spend time.

I step outside the entrance to the supermarket and turn left and walk a few steps so that I can see the tiny bungalow on Glengarry Avenue into which my family moved as part of the Jewish exodus from Toronto's densely populated downtown core. Our former home is one of only two bungalows left on Glengarry, a street dominated by monster houses. My former house, too, is destined for teardown, but at this moment it still stands as a shrine to my childhood with its broad-branched maple on the front lawn. There was a pear tree in the back, a fragrant arched rose trellis, and huge pink and white peonies on which ants marched assiduously back and forth, attracted to the buds' sweet resin. That was my first garden, and I surprise myself wondering if the garden Marie and I planted in the front of our own house last spring may be my last. It's a fleeting worry, with no medical proof thus far to give it solidity, yet there it is.

I look around the plaza and note how many of the stores bear unfamiliar names, yet it is the same plaza that I walked through as a boy of six, two steps ahead of my mother and my little sister.

From six to sixty in the blink of an eye.

Thursday, March 18

Cloudy. Bone-chilling damp. In Ontario, the month of March engenders impatience. You want winter to be done, but the season is tenacious and holds on, reminding you that warm weather, when it comes, will have something of the miraculous about it.

I arrive at the ultrasound clinic half an hour ahead of my scheduled appointment in the hope that I will be taken early. I'd been fretting since the day of my checkup, and a subsequent call to Sid, who reassured me that "it" was likely "nothing serious," failed to calm my nerves. I had spent some of my time scouring the Internet for causes of a swollen spleen, and nothing I came across seemed too disconcerting. Other than the occasional episode of atrial fibrillation, a common irregular heartbeat, I am in good health. And there are no hereditary markers to suggest the possibility of cancer. No one in my immediate family has the disease. My parents are in their mid-eighties and fully functioning. My sister and brother are in excellent health. None of my four deceased grandparents had to deal with malignancies. My parents come from large families: my mother had eight siblings, my father five. I have close to forty first cousins. One of the uncles on my mother's side has, in his old age, prostate cancer. Not so unusual. One of my many cousins has colon cancer. Given my genetic odds, I am fairly sure that I will live out my life cancer-free. I think this even though I've recently read an article by a research doctor pointing out that after the age of fifty our DNA becomes unpredictable. After fifty, he suggests, we all operate on an equal playing field called Uncertainty.

There is another, less rational reason for my feeling that cancer is unlikely. Six years ago, Marie was diagnosed with breast cancer. What are the odds of a husband and wife both being stricken with the most dreaded disease? It happens more often than one would imagine. A parent, a child. A baby can be born with a malignancy. There are households that live under a cancer cloud.

8

The ultrasound clinic is in the basement of a medical building. I sit on an uncomfortable hard-backed chair in the waiting room and take in the low ceilings, the indoor/outdoor carpeting, and the slime-green walls that are in need of painting. The technician who glances at her clipboard and calls my name is tall and middle-aged, her blonde hair perfectly straight and unusually long for a woman her age. There is no name tag on her white lab coat, though her accent suggests to me that she is Polish. She possesses the world-weary demeanour that I associate with East Europeans. I lie down on the examining table and attempt to make small talk, but she doesn't respond; she is concentrating on her screen where the images of my internal organs are about to show up and she doesn't want to invite distraction. The room is dimly lit, like a movie theatre before it is thrown into total darkness for the feature film. The technician apologizes for the coldness of the lubricant she spreads over my abdomen and then asks me to breathe in deeply and hold my breath. She repeats the instructions in the same flat voice several times. For a moment I forget the code of silence and attempt to lighten the ambiance by telling her that my years of practising yoga have prepared me for this deep breathing, but she doesn't crack a smile. Her intensity has the effect of making me question my comment: I have to ask what all the years of yoga and jogging, all those games of squash, have done for me, since here I am, lying on this table in a twilit room with some as yet indeterminate health problem, wincing as the cold scanner glides over my skin, probing what lies beneath.

8

Unless I close my eyes—and I do not want to close my eyes—I have to focus on something, so I stare at the oversized plastic eyeglass frames my technician is wearing. I haven't seen frames like those since the early 1970s. Perhaps they are back in fashion. Perhaps she has held onto them all these years. And her hairstyle—that is from the early 70s too. I surmise that her job—scrutinizing a monitor screen for deadly lesions or for potential birth defects in pregnant women—has reinforced her sombre world view. Fashion appears to mean little to her in the face of life and death. I watch carefully as her pale blue eyes narrow, and then widen, and then narrow again behind the oversized lenses. Once you enter the land of the sick you become tremendously alert to the eyes of technicians and doctors. You try your best to discern your future from those shifting orbs.

"Lean on your left side and breathe in," she instructs coldly. "Now lean on your right." She presses the scanner down repeatedly on my left side, the side that stopped Sid in his tracks. After twenty minutes she is done and tells me she is leaving the room to speak with the radiologist but will return shortly. In less than a minute the radiologist bursts into the room, one step ahead of her. He is a short, bearded man; he must have thrown on his white lab coat hastily, since it is unbuttoned and one side of the collar is standing up. He wears a black skullcap and looks tired: I think of a Yeshiva student who has been up late studying for exams. While the technician watches, he repeats parts of the ultrasound procedure, but very quickly, very deftly. The technician points to something on the screen and he shakes his head and murmurs "No, that's nothing." There is urgency to his movements and both he and the technician are quietly agitated.

"What is it?" I ask when he tells me the test is complete.

"You'll be notified by your doctor." He gives me clearance to leave, and as I sit up on the examination table in a state of mute numbness, he moves briskly to shoo me out of the room. I present a threat. He and his efficient technician know that if I linger I will start asking questions. But they are not going to be the ones to give shape to the danger I sense, to the fear settling upon me. They will not deliver the distressing message. They are the finders, not the conveyers. The job of informing will be left to my family doctor. Do doctors have a special name for that period between the moment of finding and the moment of disclosing? In my case, the scene is dramatic and absurd. I am in a room with two complete strangers who have information that will radically alter my life as well as the lives of those around me, and that knowledge is being adamantly kept from me. It is too hot to share.

But I am a newcomer to the land of the seriously sick and I have yet to learn its protocols.

"What is it?" I press the radiologist. "A tumour?"

The word leaps out of my mouth. I am hoping against hope that this God-fearing radiologist will come back with "No, no, nothing like that," but what he mutters is what he has already stated: that my family doctor will notify me. Perhaps there is no need for him, or his restrained technician, to be direct. Perhaps they have already given me, in body language, what I need to know. From the moment "tumour" is out of my mouth, it seems to me exceptionally real. Palpable, to use a medical term.

When I get home I phone Sid's office. He calls me back in a matter of minutes. I tell him that I sensed, from the reaction of the radiologist, that something was terribly wrong and would he mind getting the results as soon as possible. I tell him that I am "on *shpilkes*." Just as "tumour" had leapt out of my mouth, so does this Yiddish word for "pins and needles." I rarely use Yiddish. I am drawing—in a time of urgency—on ancestral resources. I am returning to my grandfather's tailor shop on College Street and to the Yiddish he and his fellow workers employed to talk of their daily troubles over the incessant hum of their sewing machines. I believe that the word, rooted as it is in our shared historical experience, will hasten Sid in his task.

It takes only twenty minutes for Sid to phone back with the results, twenty minutes spent pacing by the kitchen telephone, while Marie, who has already been through the wringer with her own cancer, stands next to me. I pick up the receiver. Sid, in an unfaltering voice, tells me the ultrasound shows a large mass—15.5 centimetres, a little over six inches—on my left kidney. He might have said "very large" or "extraordinarily large," since that in fact is the case. He tells me it appears to be encapsulated—that is, it doesn't seem to have spread.

"It is most likely malignant and will have to be cut out," he informs me. "And then you will move on with your life."

"And what if the cancer *has* spread?" I immediately ask. I know from what we went through with Marie that an ultrasound does not rule out metastasis.

"Don't go there," Sid responds. He is reminding me to take it one step at a time, to stop my imagination from running to catastrophe. But once you've begun your passage in the land of illness it is difficult, unreasonable even, to put a cap on your darkest speculations. I know too that by asking him about the possible spread I am asking about the apprehension of death. For up until now I, like most of us, have peered at death from a comfortable distance. It has been an abstraction. Who except the seriously ill takes hold of death with any degree of immediacy? Who gets in close to smell its sour breath? Soldiers. Police and paramedics. A select number of priests and rabbis. Those few doctors who have gone beyond their scientific training and no longer perceive death as an embarrassment.

Saturday, March 20

Sid acts swiftly. My ultrasound was performed on Thursday, March 18, and I'm booked for an appointment in the urological clinic, fourth floor, Princess Margaret Hospital, Canada's premier cancer centre, for Monday at 10 a.m. You can't do better than that. The receptionist who had called to give me my appointment told me my family doctor termed my case "an emergency." I have to agree. In the days after hearing the news, Marie and I spend hours in front of the computer screen, learning as much as we can about renal-cell carcinoma, commonly called kidney cancer. Certain people, in times of trouble, feel the need to go to the literature, read and learn. Knowledge provides a sense of control at a time when you feel helpless. After Marie was diagnosed with breast cancer, I walked with her from the hospital to The World's Biggest Book Store and bought several books on breast cancer. That evening, we sat in bed and together began our crash course on various forms of the disease. We learned that there are estrogen-positive and estrogen-negative tumours. We learned that the more aggressive tumours are HER-2 positive and that the drug Herceptin could be used against them. Marie's biopsy hadn't revealed those characteristics; we had to wait for her lumpectomy to know its nature.

In Marie's case, there had been a long foreboding about the illness. Her father had died young of pancreatic cancer. John Goldstein was a hard-working Romanian immigrant who'd survived the war in Europe and worked his way up from produce packer for IGA to supervisor of their produce department. Later he opened his own little fruit-and-vegetable shop on Eglinton Avenue. He would rise at 3 a.m. to be first in line at the Ontario Food Terminal, where he'd get first dibs on the freshest strawberries, cherries, and lettuce. He'd load his truck and bring the goods back to the store where he, his wife, Sylvia, and her parents, Moses and Ethel, would clean and wash the produce before putting it up on the stands. They opened the store at 8 a.m. and often worked until 7 p.m. That meant a sixteen-hour workday for John Goldstein. The family lived in a small one-bedroom apartment above the store. The hard work paid off. The tiny shop on Eglinton grew into a chain of eight exclusive stores that promised the finest fruits and vegetables. When John was forty-eight he complained of digestive problems and was operated on for what he thought was a bleeding ulcer. In fact it was a malignant stomach tumour. He was never told. The family along with the surgeon decided it would be too difficult for him to hear the news, a common approach in those days. The attitude persists in some parts of Eastern Europe where it is believed that mention of the word cancer might hasten the patient's demise. The John Goldstein I knew (and I knew him for six years) could have handled that news. Ten years later, when he was fifty-eight and just starting to slow down the pace of his gruelling work schedule and enjoy the fruits of his labour, he fell ill. In April 1979 he complained he didn't quite feel himself; in late May he turned jaundice. Three weeks later he was gone. I have a clear memory of walking with him and Marie through the corridor of North York General Hospital. He still had a head of thick, curly black hair. Always a smart dresser, he wore an Yves Saint Laurent bathrobe over his hospital gown. He told us during that walk that he did not regard his illness as a punishment. Knowing John, I knew that he meant it. He was a clear-thinking, hard-nosed businessman. It seemed to us that the chemotherapy they administered back then hastened his end. His spent his last day in a delirium, calling out names and half-sentences. It was heartbreaking.

John was not the only one in his family who was cancer prone; so were his immigrant cousins. Two died of the disease at the age of sixty. John's mother had died young, but John was always vague about the cause. This genetic susceptibility on her father's side weighed heavily on Marie, so I'd try to reassure her with the thought that she might take after her mother, whose parents, Moses and Ethel Donnenfeld, both lived to ninety. They outlived John by ten years.

Marie was extremely close to them all. She and John and Sylvia and Ethel and Moses comprised a post-Holocaust immigrant family; for them, closeness ensured survival. That first night after hearing her lump was malignant, Marie woke up at 2 a.m. and told me that she felt her father and grandparents were calling her to join them. I shuddered to hear her talk like that. I told her I wanted her to hang around a while longer and then I held her and told her that things would work out all right. How did I know that? I didn't, and I felt dishonest saying it, but in the weeks and months that followed I couldn't stop myself from saying it.

8

As we read through various websites devoted to renal-cell carcinoma, we come to realize that the most disconcerting factor, in my case, is the size of the tumour. We learn from a doctor on

YouTube, who speaks in a dry English accent, that the prognosis for anyone with a kidney tumour over seven centimetres—mine is more than twice that size—is "quite grim." Metastasis has most likely occurred. An older website informs us that kidney cancer does not respond to chemotherapy or radiation treatment, that the metastatic mode of the disease is basically a death notice. As we read, Marie puts her hand to her forehead and says softly, "I can't believe we *both* have cancer." She has been clear of her disease for five years; her chances of long-term survival presently look much better than mine. A little more Googling, however, reveals that in 2005 pharmaceutics came up with the wonder drugs Nexavar and Sutent, which have the power to shrink tumours—even metastatic tumours in surrounding organs—holding in check, for a time at least, the spread of cancer. I wonder, with a tumour as large as mine, if such an outcome is possible. There is also the slight chance that the tumour is benign. Some kidney tumours, especially large ones, may be slow-growing, harmless elephants. It is nice to think of that possibility, but in my case I won't place money on it.

Monday, March 22

I know Princess Margaret Hospital well; it is where Marie was treated for her cancer. I had been her "caregiver," though I dislike the term. Yes, I had given Marie care and support, but I prefer to think of myself as the primary witness to her suffering and her resolve, because "witness" emphasizes how often you are aware of your helplessness in aiding the person you love. The role of witness is, in certain aspects, more excruciating than that of patient. Now it is Marie who is holding my arm and leading me into a building that I once thought of as a house of horrors. I can remember driving with my parents in the 1950s by the old Princess Margaret Hospital when it was located on Sherbourne Street. I must have been no more than eight and I recall them telling me that it was a place where people with cancer—the word was spoken in a low whisper—came to die. I remember glancing up from the car window and seeing an emaciated patient in a ghost-white hospital gown standing by the window, gazing down at the street. Cancer was synonymous with dread, with hopelessness. The disease was shameful and unclean. It was not to be discussed and if possible not even mentioned.

In 1995, PMH moved to Hospital Row on University Avenue, just south of College Street. The first time Marie and I passed through its revolving doors and entered its bustling foyer I was surprised to discover that it was not the bleak and dismal hellhole I had imagined. I was struck by its brightness, its modern interior design, and by the streams of people entering and exiting: I thought, this is the Grand Central Station of cancer care. In a short time the brightness, the modernity, the hustle of the place failed to hide the tension, the dread anticipation, and the weariness I picked up on the grey faces of my fellow patients and their loved ones, who sat opposite me on the row seating in the large, densely packed waiting rooms. I began to think of those waiting rooms as way stations en route to the purgatory of sickness: the tests and examinations, as well as the frightening revelations and treatments.

Sid had recommended me to a surgical oncologist in the urology department he'd been sending patients to for years, and I am disappointed when the highly esteemed Dr. X does not show up but instead his resident, who informs me that he will be carrying out the examination. The young resident is heavy-set and hobbles in on two canes; he wears his hair in a crewcut. I take him for the athletic sort and wonder aloud if he's on canes because of a sports-related injury. Not so, he quickly explains; he's recently had hip surgery for a rare bone disorder. He offers the name of the disorder, but it is long and complex and I quickly forget it.

"Mine is an unpleasant condition," he informs Marie and me and then, to our astonishment, adds, "but I'd rather have this than kidney cancer."

I know from previous encounters with the medical world that in the teeter-totter doctor–patient relationship dark impulses will sometimes manifest themselves unconsciously, so I don't take his insensitive comment to heart. He is obviously green, but his spontaneity and cheerfulness are winning. He presses down on my abdomen several times, feels around, and then blurts out, "I hope to God I have a family doctor as good as yours. He must have tremendous hands because I can't for the life of me feel the mass."

He explains, as I lie there staring up at the cold fluorescent lights, what I already know: that most abdominal tumours are discovered accidently during ultrasounds or CAT scans while the patient is being tested for something unrelated. Malignant growths in the pancreas, liver, and kidney often present with no symptoms; they run silent and undeclared, and when they are picked up it is often too late. He assures Marie and me that the fact that I *feel* healthy and have no symptoms bodes well for my prognosis. When I ask about the size of the tumour, he indicates that the largeness might not be a determining factor in my survival, though he does confirm, as I already know, that spread of the disease cannot be ruled out by the ultrasound. Further testing in that regard is needed as soon as possible. He gently brushes aside the notion that the tumour might be benign with a softly spoken "Unlikely."

He informs me that I will have to wait at least two weeks for my abdominal CAT scan. This is exasperating. I am there with what the receptionist concedes is "an emergency" and yet I will have to wait weeks to discover the extent of the damage. I'd learned, by advocating for Marie during her breast cancer, that when dealing with our health-care system, it is prudent to be politely assertive and, if that doesn't work, to holler. I know that Dr. X, whom I'd expected to see, is indeed at the clinic; I recognized him, from his photo on the PMH website, standing in the corridor outside the examining rooms as we were called in. He is a sliver of a man with an oversized head and large circular glasses perched on a short nose. Ant-like, I think. I ask the resident if I can speak with Dr. X and am told there is no point until the results of the CAT scan come in.

"A minute of his time," I plead.

Reluctantly, the resident stands up and shambles out of the room on his canes, leaving the door open. A minute later Dr. X appears, or, to be exact, half appears. He doesn't want to accede fully to my request to speak with him, so he stands at the door, his upper torso and head poking into the room, his lower body planted in the hallway. I ask him if there is any way that I can get my CAT scan sooner, and his response—one that I will hear over and over again like a mantra from the doctors at PMH—is that given our overtaxed health-care system, two weeks is the best he can do. I persist and eventually Dr. X tells us that while he cannot make any promises, he will instruct his nurse to see what she can do. I know from my experiences with Marie's doctors that this is his way of acquiescing to my demand without losing face. Indeed, when his nurse arrives a few minutes later, I am advised that my CAT scan is scheduled for later in the week, and I am happy to have scored a minor victory.

Scoring a victory does not change the harsh reality of my physical condition. That reality is settling in: I harbour a massive growth inside my body and cells from that growth have likely gone beyond the parameters of the tumour. My dear friend Shel Krakofsky, a general practitioner in London, Ontario, has an expression for the spread. He will phone a surgeon to whom he's referred one of his patients and ask, "Is the horse out of the barn?"

I think about the expression. It suggests that the horse has left its proper domicile and is out of control, running rampant through the countryside. Nothing can be done to contain it.

There is a related expression: *closing the barn door after the horse has bolted.*

Regretfully, sadly, frustratingly, too late.

I do not know yet whether it is too late, though the size and shape of my abdominal tumour—comparable to that of a four-month-old fetus—conjures the thought that I am pregnant with my potential death. At the same time, the young intern on canes, in his written report for Dr. X, describes me as "a well-looking gentleman ... no hematuria [blood in the urine], no pain, no lumps or bumps anywhere else in his body." Other than the abdominal mass, I am "healthy with an excellent performance status." He has also written that the "CT scan will stage for metastatic disease."

By writing that does the young intern signal that despite my good performance level, metastasis is suspected? Am I the calm before the storm?

Friday, March 26

I am provided with a set of instructions for my CT scans. At the Medical Imaging Department of PMH I am instructed to lie down on a narrow padded bed and raise my arms straight up, like a cheerleader. The bed slides back and forth through a porthole as the scanner snaps pictures of my abdomen and chest.

Testing cannot move quickly enough when your life is threatened. Ideally, my CT scans are done the afternoon of my initial visit and by now I know the extent of my disease and a date is set for surgery. But I am stuck in the bottleneck of patients attempting to enter the System. No one—not a lover, not an expectant mother—waits as intensely as a patient. The problem with waiting is that it fuels the imagination and I find myself working up catastrophic scenes of sickness and death. I construct a film of my dwindling and demise superimposing images of those whose illnesses I've witnessed. A colleague of mine, shortly after he retired from the college, found a little black dot under his toenail that turned out to be a deadly melanoma and he was gone in six months. I visited him a month before the end. He was a smaller version of his original self and his voice was a thin squeak. I was moved by his openness, his willingness to speak openly about his disease and about his struggle to find the right doctor—the doctor who would treat him not as "a case" but as a person. His tenacity and courage have remained with me, but so has the sight of his shrunken body. I dread the prospect of being seen in that way. Isn't that what any patient fears—the bodily diminishment and disfigurement?

I'm going to become a monster.

It's that, more than dying, that scares me.

Thursday, April 1

Marie and I sit with forty or so other patients in the waiting room at PMH, anxious to learn the results of the scans. An unpromising diagnosis is most likely, yet the date, April 1, prompts some loony wishful thinking on my part. I fantasize that when Dr. X walks into the examination room he is going to say, "Guess what, kiddo? Your tumour is benign." He and his intern and nurse all shout, "April Fool!"

It suddenly occurs to me that while I have a fairly realistic take on the odds, I, like any cancer patient, am hoping for a lucky break. I am holding onto the notion that I am special—that I, above all the other poor patients who wait with me for their names to be called, deserve a reprieve. One of the big shocks in getting sick is to acknowledge that you are, after all, common flesh. Susceptible and mortal. Of course you've always known that, but knowing and accepting are two different things.

While we wait I jot down notes, impressions. Writing is a potent distraction, a means of keeping my own grim thoughts at bay. "The radiant immediacy of language," one writer called it. Writing will not shrink my tumour, but words succeed in keeping me at a safe distance from all-out despair and panic. They provide me with a sound to hold onto and a path to walk. One syllable, one word, one sentence followed by another and another. The effect is steadying.

Now and then I glance over at Marie. She is a slight woman who has held onto her good looks. She is poised, soft-spoken, often deferential. People on a daily basis misjudge her because she avoids unnecessary confrontation. I, too, for many years, misjudged her. She is reading today's newspaper, or at least pretending to. We've been married for thirty years and any marriage that long is like an unwritten epic novel, the buried scenes and dialogue apparent in the glances and nods. When you live with someone a long time you think you've plumbed the depths, but when a major crisis erupts another dimension shows itself. When she was carted off for breast surgery, she gave us two thumbs up and said she'd see us soon. Later, when she underwent radiation treatments, she'd come back each day from the hospital and fight against her tiredness, struggle to stay in the game. I had never before known the extent of Marie's resolve. She became in my eyes—and this is not a word I tend to use—heroic. Now she looks up at me and forces a weary smile and I worry that this second cancer will do us in. For I already know how depleting the sickness world can be. Even the most benign hospital visit proves enervating. You return from tests and appointments psychically drained and find to your dismay that sleep is not the rejuvenator it used to be. Once you've been diagnosed it is difficult to find a way to descend into that deep, replenishing well. You sleep fitfully on the surface and awake in anguished disbelief at the fact that this calamity is undeniably yours.

8

My name is called. Marie and I enter a brightly lit corridor where I am weighed and measured for height. We are asked to wait in one of the examination rooms. The door is closed. The room has a small desk with a computer screen and three chairs: one for the doctor, one for the patient, and one for the friend or relative who has come along to hear the news. It is imperative that you have someone to hear the news in case your anxiety prevents you from hearing it accurately. You need a witness to fact-check, to confirm the reasonableness of the hope—or despair—that you will take away from your encounter. For it is the hope–despair seesaw you find yourself on once you know you're sick.

Also in the room is an examination bed and a sink with a soap dispenser. A roll of paper towels. The walls are hospital beige. There are a few health-advisory pamphlets, but otherwise no reading material to glance at while you wait impatiently. You might say the room is neutral. Or sterile.

8

I am expecting that Dr. X, the well-known surgeon to whom I was referred, will deliver the news, but again I am disappointed. It is not Dr. X who enters the room but another of his interns. I feel an impulse to protest, but I restrain myself: I'm anxious to hear the results of the scan. The young doctor, tall and extremely polite, introduces himself in an East Indian accent. As he sits down across from us, I notice that his hand, which holds the report on my condition, is shaking and I wonder if this is the first time he has ever given the news to a patient. I can picture Dr. X handing him my file and saying, "Here, see how you do with this." Does he have the shakes because he's been assigned to act as this morning's grim-news messenger-in-training?

He tells us that the CT scan confirms the size of the tumor as well as the strong likelihood (95 per cent) that it is malignant.

He tells us that my liver, pancreas, lungs, and brain are all free of the disease, *but* (here he pauses and stares down at the report) the scan shows a lytic lesion on the ninth posterior rib.

I ask what a lytic lesion is and the young man tells me it is a bone tumour.

"Well, that is worrisome," I say.

"Yes, it is," he replies.

"Worrisome" is not a word I tend to use in conversation. Am I mirroring his formality, his decorum to distance myself from the terror?

"Can you tell from the scan whether the bone tumour is definitely malignant?" I nervously ask.

He tells me they suspect it is; Dr. X's nurse will arrange for a bone scan later in the week to confirm metastasis.

The tumour-ridden kidney is on my left side; the malignant rib is on my right. Metastasis to the bones means that the cancer cells have proliferated throughout my entire body. They are in my bloodstream.

The intern asks if I have recently injured my rib (I haven't), since that might show up as a lesion. He asks if I have experienced pain in my rib area. When cancer cells metastasize to the bone, they eat away at the surface, leaving small holes such as those made by termites in wood. I report that I have not felt pain. I ask him which rib is affected and he walks around to the back of my chair. I stand and lift my shirt. He counts up from my bottom rib until he hits the ninth and rubs his fingers there.

"It doesn't hurt," I murmur hopefully.

He shrugs his shoulders and sits down again and begins to describe the surgery I will have. Since the growth is massive, Dr. X will make a large incision down my left flank; my spleen will likely be removed; the entire kidney and its tumour will be excised. Then he will remove the cancerous portion of the rib.

The intern is speaking precisely and quickly. I note that his hand is still shaking. He wants to be done with this, and who can blame him? To hear such news is traumatic; to deliver it must likewise be distressing. I don't feel overly agitated. I have the ability, in certain stressful situations, to step outside of myself; I become, as it were, disembodied. I am listening as if from a distance to the intern's harrowing words, and when he is done I ask if I can see Dr. X. This intern is only too happy to flee the room and fetch him. A moment later Dr. X appears. I have no faith in this man. He has been practising for many years. He must know how momentous it is to hear such a diagnosis and yet he lacked the sensitivity and the courage to impart the news himself. He sent a surrogate. I require a doctor who is braver and more considerate, a doctor willing to confront my disease and my despair. As before, Dr. X does not enter the room. Not even when I have been served distressing news. He stands in the doorway, telling me we must get a bone scan scheduled as soon as possible.

"The good news," he says, "is that the lungs and brain are not affected."

This, he seems to believe, is consolation. The moment he is gone, as in a carefully staged play, his nurse sweeps into the room with a booklet on how to prepare for kidney surgery, a consent form that I am to sign, and a page listing important phone numbers: hers, the chaplain's, the hospital psychologist's. As she speaks, I hear weeping and I turn to my left. Marie sits with her forehead buried in her hands and is murmuring that she can't believe this is happening. She lifts her tear-stained face and tells the nurse that six years ago she was diagnosed with breast cancer. Now it is the nurse whose eyes begin to well up: it turns out that she too is a breast cancer survivor and feels for the two of us. I do not say a word. I do not cry. I am aware that I am not crying, even though I have the greatest reason to do just that.

Is this male bravado?

(Me strong. Me brave.)

Is it writer's detachment?

(The disembodied observer.)

Or am I grappling with the realization that I am now a member of the cancer club, the death watch?

Once the commiseration between Marie and the nurse is over, we are left to pick ourselves up and walk down the brightly lit corridor, taking this hard knowledge home with us while waiting for further instructions regarding my next test (a bone scan) and surgery. Marie has taken my arm in hers. Out of the corner of my eye, I see our nurse whispering into Dr. X's ear and pointing in our direction. She must be suggesting that he speak with us, for unexpectedly he pipes up, "Wait, you two," and asks that we follow him into a consultation room with a large table and several chairs. He wants us to know that things are not as bad as they might appear: the cancerous kidney will be removed, and the bone tumour has not been confirmed as malignant.

"And what if it is?" I ask.

"We'll remove it. There are new wonder drugs that deal effectively with metastatic kidney cancer," he replies.

He tells me that once the results of the bone scan come in, he will meet with the other members of the Tumour Board—a group of surgeons and oncologists who discuss the more complex cases and decide on best treatments. He wonders aloud whether it might be advisable to use some new drugs to shrink the tumour prior to surgery, since it is so large. He will present this option to the board. And he promises to phone me the moment he has the results of the bone scan.

What do you do after hearing that your cancer has spread to your bones? Drive home, crawl into bed, and pull the comforter over your face? What I suggest to Marie is that we drive to the Hope Street Café, one of our favourite eateries, where you sit on low chairs and tables next to leaded-pane windows. The lighting is soft, the walls and posts are of dark wood. There's a womblike closeness that feels protective. I order a savoury ham-and-cheese omelette with sweet-potato fries, and rich coffee tinged with cinnamon. Marie, ever faithful to her health regime, orders a Greek salad.

I don't know if I am in shock or in denial, but I don't feel terribly down. Marie nods when I tell her this. "That's good," she says. "We're not jumping to conclusions until all the tests are in." But it's not hope that is buoying me. Maybe it's having confirmation of what I feared. There is a settling in that comes once you know the nature of the beast, a resolve that takes over once you embrace the reality, no matter how awful. In any event, I'm not being inauthentic; I'm not hiding my pain and fear, though I know that sickness does invite all sorts of cover-ups. The patient doesn't want to overload others with the burden of his illness; the patient wants to preserve a healthy self-image and is reluctant to see himself as damaged goods. But I don't feel as though I'm putting on a front. It's more like a quiet defiance, a sort of "damn the cancer, let's savour the fries." I am surprised by my level-headedness, my equilibrium, since I had expected, on hearing such news, an emotional flood.

We make it a ritual to drive to the Hope Street Café after our appointments at PMH. I like the name "Hope Street": it's an antidote to the bureaucracy and anonymity implicit in Hospital Row, the name given to the stretch of hospitals on Toronto's University Avenue. When you are ill, you are always secretly hoping that things will turn out better than you expect. But it is good to temper your hopefulness. The year before my diagnosis I'd completed a book about various authors who had written under duress and I recalled the words of the Russian writer Varlam Shalamov: "Hope is slavery." He survived seventeen years at Kolyma, Stalin's harshest and most notorious gulag camp, located in the far reaches of northeastern Siberia, and attributed his survival, in part, to ridding himself of delusions, to refusing to hold out hope for escape or exoneration. He became a masterful practitioner of stoicism and a keen observer of camp life, composing trenchant, unforgettable stories of the lives of the men and women he knew who endured the ultimate deprivations. In the end—and out of the blue, as it were—he was granted a reprieve.

Monday, April 5

Three days after my diagnosis, I go for my bone scan at Toronto General Hospital, which is across the road from PMH. The prep for a CT scan requires the patient to drink a hideous-tasting potion served in a large milkshake cup; for the bone scan you are instructed to show up three hours early so that a nuclear tracer called radionuclide can be injected into your veins. Then you go off and drink several jugs of water to eliminate any excess tracer from your body. When you return at your allotted time, the lab technician—in my case a talkative guy in jeans and a black T-shirt, his left arm tattooed with a grinning serpent—asks you to remove jewellery and empty your pockets of any metal objects.

"That includes guns," he says grinning.

I laugh. Not because I find the joke funny but because he expects that reaction and there is no sense in ruffling the feathers of those who are treating you.

In truth, I am terrified.

The day after receiving my diagnosis—the day after sitting calmly in the womblike comfort of the Hope Street Café—all of my ribs began to burn. The question of bone pain, put to me by the tall intern as he gently rubbed my ninth posterior rib, seems to have had a suggestive effect and I am now alarmingly convinced that the malignancy has invaded all the bones of my torso. When I sit down to eat it is my left rib cage that hurts; when I lie down to sleep, it is the right. I grow more and more convinced, as the day of the scan approaches, that my bones are riddled with cancer. This is not the emotional deluge I had expected. This is the interminable gnawing anxiety that manifests itself in quirky imagined pain, mixed with sudden bursts of panic.

Reading the CT scan report, a copy of which was given to me by Dr. X's nurse, does not help: *There is a large heterogeneously enhanced mass arising from the cortex of the posterior mid pole of the left kidney and extending superiorly with dimensions of 11.7 x 15.0 cm (image 93 of series 7) x 15.9 cm in craniocaudal dimension (image 59 of series 13). The mass is displacing the kidney medially and anteriorly. It abuts the pancreatic tail and displaces the spleen superiorly.* I have no idea what "craniocaudal" means, but the mammoth size of the tumour is convincingly present in cold medical terminology and precise, irrefutable measurements. What alarms me isn't the second-last statement—*Note is made of a separately dictated chest CT report which described a lytic bone lesion in the posterior right ninth rib*—since I'd already been informed of that. Rather, the concluding statements are the ones that are most unsettling, since they provide information that neither the intern nor Dr. X had mentioned: *There are two very small ill-defined areas within the liver which are too small to characterize. We recommend follow-up of these areas on the patient's next re-staging study.* Did they not want to overload me with bad news? Is an incipient form of the renal-cell cancer there in my liver, showing up as "small, ill-defined lesions," waiting to spread?

Sickness can't help but make you crazy and the craziness becomes part of your condition. No matter how many times I explain to myself that the liver lesions are most likely nothing and that the tall intern, as well as the insensitive Dr. X, had no good reason to hide anything from me, I remain unconvinced. No matter how many times I tell myself that my rib pain is imaginary ("Think of when you started to notice it," I remind myself), it will not go away. As I lie on my sofa practising the relaxation exercises that Marie and I learned shortly after she was diagnosed with breast cancer—tensing muscles and then relaxing them while breathing and exhaling deeply—I wonder how I will manage to cope with the physical disease if I can't get my mind back in order.

8

The tattooed technician positions me on the X-ray couch and I am passed under the porthole-shaped scanner while the gamma camera zaps images of my entire skeleton. My ribs hurt more than ever as the camera surveys my bones for signs of treason. If the signs are there, they will show up as dark splotches radiologists call "hot spots." I can see them on the X-rays of the shrunken skeletons that line the walls of the lab.

They remind me of the tiny skeletons hung from porch railings on Halloween to frighten children.

"Are you sure your left kidney hasn't already been removed?" the technician asks as he stares at a computer screen.

"Quite sure," I say, and wonder why he asks. Has my tumour obliterated his view of the kidney?

"Have you ever had any serious bone injuries?"

"None," I respond.

His questions increase my anxiety; it becomes apparent to me why technicians are instructed to exchange little more than courtesies. Since being diagnosed I am hyper-attentive. Every gesture and every inflection of the voices of those who treat me are ripe for interpretation. I search for clues as to how my cancer story is going to proceed. The craziness I am experiencing is partly a question of control: I recognize that I have only a minor role to play in determining the plot of my illness narrative. The primary author is the disease itself, writing its tale on the cells of my body. The doctors are the powerful interpreters, as they have the expertise to read the signs. But I can reclaim my humanity by writing my own narrative, focusing on my reactions, my expectations and fears. I can affirm my identity by acting as an honest witness to my own suffering.

The scan is complete, and the technician informs me that I can get dressed and leave. He makes no more jokes. He's grown quiet staring at the computer screen, checking the quality of the pictures he has taken. As I slide off the table, he says, "Good luck!" and I wonder why he is wishing me luck. No other technician has ever done so. Does he feel that I, especially, will need it?

8

Thus far I have told no one of my cancer. I carry on, tight-lipped. Why am I reluctant to speak of my condition?

Is it because I was raised in an environment of duplicity and cover-up? (Wear a mask. Do not let anyone know your true thoughts or feelings. Hide weakness. If others sense you are wounded they will pounce.)

Is it because sharing my news will invite trespass and I wish to avoid being reduced to an anecdote? (My status as well-regarded poet, essayist, and teacher downgraded to "poor patient.")

Is it because once the news is out I will be forced to contend with the emotional reactions of others? (Their disbelief. Their pity. Their wariness. Their over-concern.) I need to focus my attention on the task at hand. Which is what? Coping with my new life: the tests, the doctors, the unknown.

Am I reluctant to share my news because I am ashamed to have cancer? (I am a loser in the eyes of others?)

Or because I am shocked into silence by the sheer enormity of my disease? ("Thou hast brought me unto the dust of death," cries the poet of Psalm 22:15. "My tongue cleaveth to my mouth.")

Or because speaking of my condition makes it all too real?

8

I have to tell my two children, Justine and Adam. They are adults and already sense something is up when they listen to my voice on the telephone. I feel lousy about having to tell them. They have already suffered with one sick parent, but to my surprise they greet the news with measured concern. I wonder whether they appreciate the seriousness of my condition, or whether they assume that because Marie came through, so will I. Perhaps they mute their worry so as not to agitate me. I am easily agitated.

Soon the stress of knowing that I am seriously ill interferes with my teaching and student appointments, makes my attendance erratic enough that I am forced to reveal my condition to those who need to know.

When I phone Yael Katz, my dean at the college, to notify her of my condition, I obfuscate. I tell her I am ill, but I am vague. I cannot bring myself to say the word "cancer." I announce that I am going to retire from the college for medical reasons. She, of course, is surprised by the news. An hour later I phone her again and confess the details of my kidney tumour. When I pronounce the word "cancer" the very sound of it is shocking to my ears. Is it really me who has been so singled out and marked?

Yael rises to the occasion. She is empathetic and suggests that I take sick leave to deal with my medical matters. My thinking has been so muddled that I hadn't even considered sick leave as an option, but it is the right path since it will give me time to work on my illness. In one of my favourite books, *A Short History of Decay*, the caustic philosopher E.M. Cioran states: "The man suffering from a characterized sickness is not entitled to complain: he has an occupation." I spend a good portion of each day on the phone with various medical departments arranging for tests and, once they are done, trying to obtain the results. Or I revise the poems I am putting together for a new collection until the thought of cancer cells proliferating in my bloodstream stops me cold. I call out to Marie and we talk and sometimes hug each other and weep. Or I talk with my son, Adam, who works as a studio manager for a prominent New York City fashion photographer; Adam has tremendous wit and always manages to make me smile with outrageous stories of the New York fashion industry. Or I enjoy a brief noontime visit from our daughter, Justine, who is a lawyer for the Children's Aid Society. She is in family court three days a week arguing to take children away from abusive parents. The court is a five-minute drive from our house. She lifts my spirits with stories of her twin sons, Aiden and Jacob. I recently bought my twin grandsons ukuleles and while they can't pluck notes yet, they strum along with me as I play songs for them on my guitar. Sometimes, after my daughter leaves, I think of the possibility that I may not be present for the boys in the years ahead and that usually leads to a few bad hours.

Tuesday, April 6

Passover: my favourite Jewish holiday on account of the grand and universal theme of liberation. When I was a small boy, the Seder—the ritual Passover dinner and service—was held at my grandparents' house on Baldwin Street, where we were joined by numerous aunts, uncles, and cousins. My earliest recollection is crunching a tasteless piece of *matzoh*—Passover's flat, unleavened bread—and sticking my baby finger in the syrupy kosher wine as we recited the ten plagues that God inflicted upon the Egyptians in response to Pharaoh's unwillingness to set the people of Israel free. I was admonished, from a young age, not to lick my pinky after dipping it into the wine cup, as that would infer that I enjoyed the pain of others. Vanquish your enemies, but do no gloat over their destruction. Surely there was something else I noted as we recited the plagues: that pestilence comes as retribution from God. Was that my earliest apprehension of disease—that it comes as a punishment?

Though Marie and I are stressed over my diagnosis, we decide to go ahead with our plan to host a Seder that includes Adam, who has flown in from New York, Justine and her husband, Michael, our grandchildren, as well as Michael's parents. It's incumbent upon the youngest child at the Seder to ask, "Why is this night different from all other nights?" and that fundamental question sparks the Exodus story of Moses and Pharaoh and all that ensued. But for me, having just been diagnosed with a deadly disease, the crucial question is framed not as "Why is this night different from all other nights" but "Why is this Passover different from all other Passovers?" And the answer for me is that this Passover I have been diagnosed; this Passover the Angel of Death did not *pass over* my house as he was supposed to. In Egypt, the Jews had been instructed to place the blood of the Paschal lamb on their doorposts so that the Angel of Death would know who dwelled within and would dutifully pass by. He was on a lethal mission, executing what God had laid out for the tenth plague: the death of the Egyptian first-born males. I am a first-born male, but why the mix-up? My house is appropriately marked with the *mezuzah* Jews are commanded to place on the doorpost, a hearkening back to the identifying lamb's blood. To be fair, I have to remind myself that the Angel of Death didn't exactly visit me on Passover: he merely left a calling card with a note saying, "Sorry I missed you; catch you later."

Passover is a holiday that takes you from suffering to deliverance, and now that I am afflicted, the theme of deliverance resonates ever more powerfully. The journey out of bondage is conveyed not only through the narrative of Exodus but through the symbolism of the food we eat: the salt water in which we dip our hard-boiled eggs reminds us of the tears of our people; the horseradish brings to mind the bitterness of their lives. Chopped nuts, grated apples, cinnamon, and sweet red wine are combined to form a mixture called *charoset*, which represents the mortar used by our distant ancestors to build the Egyptians' storehouses and pyramids. Because we once were slaves and now are free, it is our duty on the night of Passover to enjoy as royalty might. Hence, the overabundance: gefilte fish, followed by chicken soup with matzoh balls, followed by salad and brisket and not one but two different chicken dishes; and all of this accompanied by tsimmis (a stew of carrots, sweet potatoes, apples, and prunes), potato kugel (pudding), and of course kosher pickles.

I have brought my guitar to the Seder table, and after we finish our meal and say our concluding prayers I pass around the lyrics to Peter, Paul and Mary's 1963 rendition of "Tell It on the Mountain," a reworking of an African-American spiritual dating back to the mid-1800s. The famous trio had turned the original song, which celebrated the birth of Jesus, into an anthem for the civil-rights movement by appropriating the narrative and imagery of Exodus. As I strum the three simple chords that comprise this many-layered hymn to freedom, I forget my disease. Or rather my disease is taken up into a tapestry of suffering that includes the Jews of Exodus, African-American slaves, and Yeshua of Nazareth, my crucified Jewish brother. The bodies of the first-born of Egypt are in the tapestry as well, along with their wailing mothers and fathers.

Friday, April 9

Dr. X would have received the results of my bone scan the day after the test but he has not called with the results. I wonder, given the rigidity of our health-care system, if it would be possible to change doctors. I would like to find a doctor who will not abandon me. But I wonder, too, given the seriousness of my condition and the pressing need for surgery, whether it is wise to spend time running after another surgeon. Dealing with an illness requires tremendous psychic energy, and then you find that you have to muster additional reserves to navigate your way through the thick bureaucracy of the health-care system. After repeated calls to Dr. X's office from both Marie and me, we try his nurse, the one who commiserated with us on April Fool's Day. It is a Friday, four days since I've had the scan. If I do not hear from Dr. X today, I will have to wait out the weekend and that will be excruciating. His nurse returns our morning call at noon, telling me that Dr. X is extremely busy. She promises to speak with him and she is true to her word, for late in the afternoon he calls.

"I have good news and bad news," Dr. X says. His voice is more jovial than usual and for a moment I imagine that his line is the lead-in to a Borscht Belt joke.

"The bad news is that the tumour on your rib is malignant. The good news is that the rest of your bones are clear."

Dr. X reminds me that the Tumour Board has yet to discuss my case. He is not sure whether the best approach is to begin treating me with a chemotherapeutic drug before surgery in order to shrink the tumour and stop the spread of the

cancer or to go ahead and operate. He will get in touch once
the board has come to a decision.

Despite the confirmation that I have metastatic kidney
cancer, I am relieved. I was convinced that the bone scan would
show so many hot spots that Dr. X would tell me it's game over
and no point operating, since the chances of survival are slim.

Now that the parameters of my disease have come into
focus, the soreness in my ribs begins to subside, and as it does
I wonder whether my pain was due to the stress of not knowing how far the cancer had spread; as a patient you quickly
learn that it's the not-knowing that is hardest to bear. At least
now I am certain of what I am dealing with. There are still
many things about my disease I cannot know until surgery
is performed and my tissue analyzed. And then there will be
more unknowns down the road: How will I respond to treatments? Will my cancer recur?

§

Uncertainty.

It is uncertain that the plane we board will take us safely
to our destination. It is uncertain that the fetus developing in
the womb will be born healthy. It is uncertain that when we do
something so ordinary as lie down to sleep, we will awake. That
is why religious Jews upon awaking recite the prayer *Modeh
Ani:* "I give thanks, living and eternal King, for you have mer-
cifully restored my soul within me." The patient with a serious
illness, whether he believes in God or not, understands the
impetus for such prayer. The patient with a serious illness cannot forget that our existence is tenuous, our fate uncertain.

§

It may well be that our shame regarding sickness and our
embarrassment over death have prevented us from developing
a language commensurate to the discussion of these matters.
We risk tactless comments, miscommunications, good inten-
tions gone awry. Some cancer conversations prove to be easier

than others. When I phone my brother Randy, who has lived in Tampa for thirty years, and tell him the details, he is in disbelief. Randy is ten years younger than I, the baby in our family. He is a successful businessman, a man of action. The day after hearing the news, he rebounds from the shock and calls with the telephone number of a close friend's father who is a kidney-cancer survivor. Randy urges me to call him to talk about my own situation. He also has the number of a friend's uncle, a urological oncologist at the Mayo Clinic. I can call him any time I like, Randy says. This is what I need: practical help. But I'm not able to extrapolate from this encounter with my brother and trust that by telling people about my condition I will receive more help. For various reasons, I remain closed, suspicious. And perhaps I am right to feel guarded, for other conversations do not go as well. One relative weeps on the phone when I reveal my condition. Her weeping goes on and on. She cannot catch her breath to speak. What does the weeping mean to me? I have two reactions. One: This is the sort of weeping one offers the dead. Two: The longer the weeping goes on, the more it seems that this encounter is about her. The ex-husband of my sister hears of my condition through the grapevine; I haven't heard from him in twenty years, yet he calls to commiserate. But he has no gift for empathy and our conversation is bizarre, awkward, just the sort of encounter I had feared.

8

My brother is not the only solid support we rely on. My good friend Shel Krakofsky, a family physician and fellow writer, helped us get through Marie's breast cancer and has been talking with me since Sid discovered the growth. Shel lives in an old farmhouse near the small town of Komoka, which is just outside of London, Ontario. Few have heard of Komoka and even fewer of George "Mooney" Gibson, who is buried there. Gibson, a major-league catcher, was part of the Pittsburgh Pirates team that won the 1909 World Series against Ty

Cobb's Detroit Tigers. "Four games to three," Shel, who is an avid baseball fan, will tell you. He likes to drive his guests to see Mooney's grave.

When I told Shel my renal-cell carcinoma diagnosis he was cautiously reassuring. "It might be a slow-growing cancer," he suggested. "And if it *has* metastasized the new wonder drugs will likely render it a chronic, not a fatal, condition."

Coincidentally, Shel's daughter, Rivka, represents a company that distributes Sutent (sunitinib malate), one of those miracle drugs used to control kidney cancer. When Rivka hears of my tumour, she calls to let me know that the country's first-ever patient/doctor conference on kidney cancer is being held in Toronto on April 10, this coming weekend. I immediately go to the Kidney Cancer Canada website and sign up to attend the conference. Taking this action provides some relief. My condition is urgent and I desperately want to do something to help myself, yet I've been placed in a state of suspended animation, waiting for the Tumour Board—for me, the name has a Kafkaesque ring—to meet and discuss the best path of treatment. I fantasize that cancer cells are proliferating at an alarming rate, invading other areas of my body. Listening to the top surgeons and oncologists discuss the latest developments in treating renal-cell carcinoma is one proactive step I can take at this time. In addition, two of the doctors who sit on the Tumour Board—the oncologist Jennifer Knox and the surgeon Michael Jewett—will be speaking at the conference. I want to introduce myself to them. I want them to be able to put a face to my scans and X-rays when they come to discuss my case.

Saturday, April 10

At the conference, smiling volunteers offer me an identification tag. I am to choose from "health provider," "caregiver," or "patient." I print my name in full, peel off the back, and paste the tag to my jersey. Why do I feel uncomfortable wearing the label "patient"? This is not like the scarlet badge of shame that was imposed upon Hawthorne's Hester; it is not the yellow badge of persecution forced upon my people in the ghettos of Europe. Still, I feel marked, vulnerable. I have recently discovered, in one of the cancer books I am reading, that the root of the word "patient" is the Latin *patiens*, akin to the Greek verb πάσχειν (*paskhein*): to suffer. I do not want to be The Sufferer. I would rather be a step up in this medical caste system: The Caregiver. (That badge goes to Marie.) I envy those on the top rung, The Health Providers, the system's high priests.

Marie and I find a familiar face: Rivka is in attendance. She takes me by the arm and introduces me to Bernard, the father of a close friend. Bernard is sixty-five and has lived with metastatic kidney cancer for five years. At the time he was diagnosed he had spots on his liver and lungs. He tells me that Sutent has worked wonders, but that all the new miracle drugs are effective for only so many years. They generally ward off progress of the disease for three or four years, at which point a new drug needs to be administered to check the cancer's spread.

"You are lucky," Bernard tells me. "Had you been diagnosed ten years ago there would have been few options."

Bernard has gone through the list of available medications and now needs Afinitor, which the Ontario government will not fund. So Bernard has entered a clinical trial at Montreal's McGill University Health Centre.

"Check out the different clinical trials," he advises me, and writes on a piece of paper the URL for a website that lists them.

He also advises that I stay in shape.

"I do the treadmill and yoga. It's uplifting and lets me know that my body is still in working order."

An accountant by profession, Bernard has become an advocate for better cancer care. Rivka, who is standing by, informs me that he has appeared on television, telling his cancer story and appealing to our provincial government for more funding. All this while enduring stage IV kidney cancer.

Bernard wishes me well, and Rivka steers me to another corner of the room to meet Deb Maskens, the head of Kidney Cancer Canada, which she co-founded in 2006. Deb epitomizes The Survivor. Diagnosed with renal-cell carcinoma at the age of fourteen, she suffered a reoccurrence twenty-two years later. (Talk about rare: the majority of kidney cancer patients are male and over fifty-five years of age.) Deb has had eight major surgeries and is currently being treated with Nexavar. She has lived fourteen years with stage IV kidney cancer and looks fit. She is a warm, articulate, no-nonsense lady who leads the fight for greater government funding of cancer drugs while lending support to fellow sufferers.

8

We return to our seats and I introduce myself to the woman next to me, who also bears the Patient tag. She tells me her name is Carey. She is tall, blonde, my age. Her caregiver female friend sits next to her. I see Carey has rested her cane beside her chair. She was first diagnosed with kidney cancer twelve years ago; the disease has reappeared in her liver and spine, hence the cane. She informs me that with surgery on her spine comes the risk of damaging tissue and nerves; the doctors are considering CyberKnife, a super-exact form of radiation. She also tells me that though she has been on a strict macrobiotic diet these past twelve years, her undying love of sweets is what likely caused her reoccurrence. Something about Carey gives me the sense that she is a New Ager groping for an environmental link to her cancer, and while I do not subscribe to the idea that cancer is caused by the foods we eat I find her conviction infectious. Suddenly I'm thinking about my own love of sweets—all the butter tarts and chocolate cakes I've consumed—wondering if indeed it was sugar that morphed my cells into a malignancy.

The conference's keynote speaker is the accomplished oncologist Dr. Robert Buckman, a well-known television and radio personality. Buckman is personable, humorous, and humane. By chance, I had met him at a resort in northern Ontario some years back. A natural raconteur, he held court on the communal dock, and kept his fellow guests in stitches with his jokes and anecdotes. English by birth, Buckman was part of the same British comedy reviews that hatched the likes of the Monty Python crew. I learned of his comedic past from my doctor friend Shel, who also informed me that Buckman suffers from an autoimmune disease. That explains what I witnessed one day at the resort. I was changing to go for a swim and through the window of our cabin I watched Dr. Buckman as he walked down the dirt path to the lake. Suddenly, he stopped; he was having trouble breathing and stood for several minutes, gulping air, attempting to regroup. When the breathing got better, he ambled on toward the lake. Here was a man who, despite his own distress, devoted himself to helping others, while maintaining his sense of humour. What was that slogan the Brits used to get through the Blitz? "Keep calm. Carry on." Buckman would have added, "And while you're at it, have a good laugh."

Robert Buckman's talk, "Cancer Is a Word," is intended to deconstruct our attitude toward the most dreaded of diseases. Buckman provides the following scenario: You are out shovelling snow and have chest pains and are rushed to the hospital. There you are told you have had a mild heart attack. You ask the physician, "What are my chances of dying of future heart failure?" and are told 5 per cent. Buckman asks: "Are you mildly anxious, moderately anxious, or severely anxious?" Most in the room raise their hands for the moderately anxious category. Next scenario: A tumour is discovered and you have it removed. It is malignant. You ask the physician, "What are my chances of dying from this cancer?" and are told 5 per cent. "Are you mildly anxious, moderately anxious, or severely anxious?" Most raise their hands for severely anxious. This, Buckman believes, has to do with our fear of the word "cancer." He points out that we treat the word generically, while in fact there are over three hundred different forms of cancer, some far more lethal than others. He also illustrates how "our level of fear over cancer is commensurate with our pre-set level of anxiety." (Person A is told she has a 90 per cent chance of surviving her cancer and is relieved. Person B is given the same statistics and can't stop worrying: she's certain she'll be in the unfortunate 10 per cent who suffer an untimely death.) Buckman wants our reactions to cancer to be based on solid medical information so that we are "appropriately frightened or appropriately reassured."

Buckman's argument is sane, convincing, and I laugh along with everyone else at his jokes. But I feel that some details are missing. "Cancer" is a word. So is "Death." If you were to ask people how they want to die, most will say "quickly and painlessly": i.e., a massive heart attack. Cancer provides no rapid exit. With a cancer death, we think "slowly and painfully." The obit states, "She passed away after a long battle with cancer." Some still shy away from even mentioning cancer and euphemistically state, "after a long illness." Either way, the common denominator is "long." I'm reminded of what the Canadian poet and songwriter Leonard Cohen said in a CBC interview: "It's not death I fear; it's the preliminaries."

The next speaker, the surgeon Dr. Anil Kapoor, begins his presentation with statistics. Kidney cancer makes up only 3 per cent of all the cancers in North America. Most kidney tumours are found incidentally, through scans and ultrasounds. The vast majority are discovered in the early stage, when the tumours are small and local. Fifteen to twenty per cent are metastatic cancers. That means that, at most, only two out of ten persons at the time of diagnosis have a spread of their cancer. I look at Dr. Kapoor's coloured charts and grimace at my lousy luck. If only I had gone for an ultrasound five years earlier, the tumour might have been small and localized. But why would I have gone for an ultrasound? What indication was there that I needed one? Should everyone over fifty years of age have an ultrasound? There is a clinic downtown—Medcan—where the wealthy go for their medical care. It advertises "Executive Health." An abdominal ultrasound is part of their routine checkup. If I were an executive would my cancer have been detected sooner?

Surgeons are the rock stars of the medical world and tend to present themselves with panache. Dr. Kapoor is tall and finely suited. His hands are his most interesting feature, the long slender fingers unfolding as he makes each point. He describes, with the help of graphic slides, how a malignant kidney is removed, and then goes on to mention the astonishing costs involved. The "sandwich bag" into which the tumour is placed before it is lifted out of the body (this prevents the diffusion of cancer cells) costs $500. Sometimes the tumour is emulsified in a blender-like gizmo that runs $3,000. I'm not sure why Kapoor talks money, but I find it fascinating and grounding. It's a reminder of the cost our health-care system has to bear for each operation.

After the presentation, Dr. Kapoor entertains questions from the participants and, with the Tumour Board's forthcoming review of my case in mind, I ask if it is advisable to try to shrink a tumour with chemotherapeutic drugs before operating. Dr. Kapoor calls this "a good question," and tells his audience there are clinical trials under way to determine the effectiveness of neo-adjuvant therapy (therapy before surgery). For now, Dr. Kapoor declares, the proven way to treat a kidney tumour remains as it has been for the past hundred years: surgical removal. What has changed in recent years is the technique that surgeons employ. For instance, laparoscopic surgery, a less invasive technique in which operations are performed away from the tumour site through small incisions made elsewhere in the body.

I pay close attention to the words of the next speaker, the oncologist Dr. Mary Mackenzie from the London Regional Cancer Centre. She is speaking on advances in treating metastatic renal-cell carcinoma (that's me) and begins by stating that she is bringing "a message of progress and hope in the treatment of metastatic renal cancer." She focuses on a sixty-two-year-old male she has been treating since 2005. "Patient W," as she calls him, came to her with a large kidney tumour and several metastases to the liver. In 2005 the only drug available to treat the spread was Interferon, which Patient W self-injected three times daily. This held the cancer in check until 2006, when the first of the miracle drugs, Nexavar, came onto the market, followed shortly by Sutent and Affinitor. These drugs have kept Patient W alive and relatively well. Dr. Mackenzie tells us that Patient W likes to go south and golf, and her slide show has a close-up of a putter about to tap a golf ball. (I take it that golf represents the continuance of a successful middle-class life.) Cancer and the prescribed drugs have not interfered significantly with Patient W's lifestyle and Dr. Mackenzie hopes that she will provide him "with many more years of golf in the sun."

The rosy picture does have its downside. Dr. Mackenzie delineates the possible side effects of the wonder drugs: mouth sores, diarrhea, fatigue, as well as sensitivity to sun. I take heart to think that these drugs may keep me alive, but wince thinking of their possible impact on my health. She points out that these drugs are not effective for all parts of the body: the spread of kidney cancer to the bones (again, me) or the brain is "troublesome," and in such problematic cases radiation, which does not generally work well on renal-cell carcinoma metastases, may be attempted.

In one slide, Dr. Mackenzie pays tribute to Dr. Judah Folkman, from the Children's Hospital in Boston, who in the 1990s demonstrated that a malignant tumour could incite neighbouring blood vessels to grow around itself and thus acquire its own blood supply. Folkman called the insidious process "tumour angiogenesis." His discovery led researchers to ask what would happen if they were able to cut off the blood supply to a cancerous tumour. Wonder drugs such as Sutent and Nexavar accomplish this, and in the case of renal tumours that are particularly bloody, the results can be miraculous.

The most memorable portion of Dr. Mackenzie's presentation is a cartoon slide titled "Removing the Primary Tumour." It depicts the kidney tumour as a flying saucer with an alien's head peering out the top; Dr. Mackenzie has labelled this "the mother ship." Arrows radiate out from this mother ship to what are labelled "baby metastases," depicted as much smaller flying saucers operated by tiny aliens. According to Dr. Mackenzie, it is believed that the mother ship sends messages to the babies—once the mother ship is removed (i.e., the kidney tumour excised), the biological communication between the mother and her babies is cut off and the cancer spread is slowed or stopped altogether. If that is so, it seems to me that the Tumour Board's decision regarding my treatment should be a no-brainer: the tumour has to come out.

Dr. Mackenzie's cartoon helps me understand a complex biological process and makes its point beautifully, but I wonder about her image of alien spaceships. From the reading I have done, I know that tumours do not originate from without. Cancer is not an invasion of the body, despite the fact that some patients perceive it as such. It is self-generated. (In biological terms it is *endogenous,* not *exogenous.*) In his book *The Emperor of All Maladies: A Biography of Cancer,* Dr. Siddhartha Mukherjee, a devoted oncologist, declares that with cancer "nothing is extraneous. Cancer's life is a recapitulation of the body's life, its existence a pathological mirror of our own.... Down to their innate molecular core, cancer cells are hyperactive, survival-endowed ... inventive copies of ourselves." According to Mukherjee, tumour angiogenesis—the process that feeds my fifteen-centimetre tumour fresh blood—"exploits the same pathways that are used when blood vessels are created to heal wounds." It is startling and macabre to think that I have grown this deadly tumour myself, that my body is helping it to thrive and enlarge.

At the lunch break I introduce myself to the oncologist Dr. Jennifer Knox, a tall and neatly dressed blonde. She is standing next to Dr. Kapoor. I tell her my case will be coming before the Tumour Board and that I want her to put a human face to the reports.

Dr. Kapoor remembers me for my question regarding neo-adjuvant therapy. When I mention that the cancer has spread to my rib, he and Dr. Knox glance quickly at each other. I am attuned to glances. Is it my imagination, or do their voices drop in pitch as they concur that in a case such as mine (tending toward the hopeless?), Sutent may indeed be useful before surgery?

I swing over to the other side of the room and introduce myself to Dr. Michael Jewett. Soon after I met Dr. X, and realized that he was not the doctor for me, I spoke with the surgeon Dr. Steven Gallinger, a friend of a friend, and asked if he could recommend some surgeons specializing in kidney cancer. Jewett's name topped Gallinger's list. I find Jewett to be genial, sympathetic. I ask if he will meet me for a consultation and he hands me his card and suggests that I email him. This gives me hope. Perhaps he can shed more light on my case. Perhaps I can ask him if he will perform my surgery.

8

I am taking notes at the conference in a blue Hilroy spiral notebook. I flip through the pages. There are brief diary entries, questions to ask doctors, phone numbers of medical personnel, and observations.

Why do I keep a notebook? I began this habit of collecting quotations and jotting down thoughts in my last year of high school. Since then I have filled several spiral notebooks with reflections and found witticisms. The lines I copy out of books are those that have some relevance to my personal struggle, my ongoing project of building a self other than the self that was intended for me by my family and by my social milieu. If I go back and read early notebooks filled with these quotations, I am struck by the fact that the lines I chose remain relevant to me and that my personal quest has, in essence, not altered. Some quotations are by now so well known to me that they no longer surprise. I see myself in the familiar words. Others, that I had forgotten, impress me as much as when I first chanced upon them. The first entry in my first notebook of 1969 is from an interview Boris Pasternak gave *The Paris Review* in the fall of 1960: "One must live and write restlessly, with the help of the new reserves that life offers.... Life around us is ever changing and I believe that one should change one's slant accordingly—at least once every ten years." Lines such as these serve as equipment for living.

In the same notebook I find eerily prescient lines from German poet Heinrich Heine's "Schopfungslieder" (Creation Song):

> Disease was the most basic ground
> Of my creative urge and stress;
> Creating I could convalesce,
> Creating, I again grew sound.

Heine, and others who devote their lives to writing, believe the creative process is curative. Wallace Stevens, the great American poet, declared: "Poetry is a health." When I copied those lines by Heine into my blue notebook, I mistakenly assumed that his "disease" was a psychological disorder. Later I learned, from reading Ernst Pawel's superb biography, *The Poet Dying: Heinrich Heine's Last Years in Paris*, that the German poet suffered from what his contemporaries believed was advanced syphilis but that experts now believe was ALS (Lou Gehrig's disease). The illness exacted a heavy toll: Pawel describes the middle-aged poet as a seventy-pound skeleton nearly sightless and usually sedated. Heine passed through his season in hell producing an impressive body of powerful poetry and prose. I learn, too, that Pawel never saw his evocative biography in print. He wrote the book while suffering the final stages of lung cancer and died one year before it was published.

Throughout my several notebooks are drafts of poems and essays. This is where the reading and thinking have borne fruit and my own voice breaks through. These drafts, along with the quotations from books, interviews, and articles, form a type of self-portrait.

My current notebook—which I began when I was diagnosed—has selections from the illness narratives I am currently rereading: Harold Brodkey's *This Wild Darkness*, Anatole Broyard's *Intoxicated by My Illness*, Gillian Rose's *Love's Work*, and Donald Hall's *Life Work*. A year before I was diagnosed I completed an essay on the relationship between illness and literature called "The Angel of Disease." It was the final, and several reviewers noted, strongest essay in my collection *What the Furies Bring*. Ironically, my research on the subject of illness provided me with an adequate collection of books on the subject as well as an intellectual foundation for confronting my cancer. Of course, reading and thinking about disease is oceans apart from coping with a potentially terminal condition. Once the doctor tells you you are ill, you begin to eke out your existence as a patient. Your life becomes an improvisation around the theme of illness.

My current notebook also contains drafts of poems as well as brief diary entries that are intended to provide an accurate record of my illness. I know from experience that the poems I am drafting are too emotional to be of substance. They resonate with self-pity and hurt; they do not, as Yeats's epitaph advises, "Cast a cold eye on life, on death." Coldness is not the only means a writer can employ to distance himself from trauma. Humour will do. A snatch of doggerel that I wrote after learning of my diagnosis and that I immediately considered good only for the waste basket strikes me now as an honest evocation of my condition.

> *My tumour's the size of a football*
> *My rib has the look of Swiss cheese.*
> *Oh doctor, doctor, doctor,*
> *Won't you help me please?*
>
> *I'm waiting to hear my sentence*
> *I'm practising sick man's art.*
> *Doc, give me something to hope for*
> *And cure this patient heart.*

Spiritual illness—what some would call psychic disturbance—has most often fuelled my poetry, but there have been times when physical illness has served as my muse's agent. Since the age of forty I have endured a serious physical calamity every ten years. In the fall of my fortieth year, I awoke one morning, turned on the light, and noticed it was less bright than usual and mildly distorted. I put up with this greying vision for two days, thinking it might clear on its own, and then went to my ophthalmologist. He told me I'd suffered a venous occlusion (blocked blood vessel) in the retina of my left eye. There was bleeding, and the buildup of fluid led to a significant loss of central vision. As the poem you are about to read indicates, on my first visit to the doctor I misconstrued his medical "venous" for the classical "Venus." This mishearing rescued a medical event from the mundane and became the pivot on which the poem turned.

Venus Occluded

I awoke one morning to discover one eye
weird, blurry, as if opened underwater.
At first I thought I was imagining the effect,
denial my reaction to any physical mishap.

But two days later I found myself sitting
in the darkened chamber, the ophthalmologist
hunched over me, his miner's light probing
the flooded landscape of my retina. "There it is."
Then the ominous pause. "A venous occlusion ...
some damage ..." I understood occlusion as blockage,
but not being from the scientific side of things
or wanting, perhaps, to accept responsibility for failed
    vision
I heard him speak the name of the Goddess
and wondered if those images were fading
because they'd not been loved enough.

I had to wait five years after losing part of my vision to envisage the poem. Five years to absorb and distill and distance myself from the trauma and then to re-create the experience for others. I especially like the way in which the last lines of the poem turn on the patient's regret, and how that regret is comprehensible to anyone who has taken the wonders of each day for granted.

Ten years after my eye episode (I had recently turned fifty) I noticed, in the midst of a strenuous squash game at the YMCA, a fluttering sensation in my chest. A few weeks later, following a long swim in the Y pool, I noted my heart beating fast and erratically; it lasted only a few minutes and I wrote it off as a one-time anomaly. These instances recurred with no considerable effect until one afternoon, after running my usual five kilometres, I returned home and got into an argument with Marie over something to do with her mother or my mother, I cannot exactly recall, but it was something that at the time seemed crucial but was most likely—as with many spousal arguments—inane. My heart began pounding: I thought of a trout trying to leap from the water. I felt breathless and Marie drove me to Sunnybrook Hospital, where I was diagnosed with paroxysmal atrial fibrillation, a non-life-threatening arrhythmia of the heart.

Our medical imaging has advanced to the point where a man, mildly sedated, can watch a scope pass over and examine the furrows of his intestines; a woman can see the small limbs and beating heart of her soon-to-be-born child. During my first echocardiogram (I was having the test to rule out any structural abnormalities; there were none) I lay on an examining bed and watched a computer screen on which the chambers of my heart opened and closed. I marvelled at the rush of blood entering the chambers and at the amplified sound it made: the *swish swish* of a washing machine. The longer I observed my beating heart, the stranger and more primitive it seemed. I admired its single-mindedness but wondered about my connection to this drudge of a workhorse that plodded on and on, never questioning existence. What did this muscle have to do with the thinking and feeling me? In an attempt to lay claim to my heart, and to take account of my life, I went home after the test and wrote the first draft of my poem "Heart."

> So there you are at last,
> on the diagnostician's screen,
> fluctuating between clinical grey
> and amber, chambers
> opening and closing:
> a mollusc
> kneading its vital fluid.
>
> You look so primitive.
> Who would suspect you to inhabit
> a human chest, to fasten
> with such tenacity
> onto memories, lyrics,
> frames of an old black
> and white film?
>
> Hoarder, I lie awake at night
> hearing you *thump thump*

as if you were banging on the door
of my life, pleading
for one more chance
to wipe the slate clean
and begin again.

Sunday, April 11

The day following the conference I email Dr. Jewett to give him the specifics of my CT scan and to ask if we can meet. He emails me back, letting me know that it is best to wait until after the Tumour Board's decision to set a date for a consultation. I am relieved that he acknowledges my email. I am feeling lonely, abandoned, and Jewett's willingness to respond gives me hope. It is nearly one month since Sid discovered my tumour. On the day he received the ultrasound report he told me I needed an operation ASAP, yet I find the PMH process bewilderingly sluggish. How long after the Tumour Board's decision before I hear from Dr. X? How long after that before some action is taken?

Tuesday, April 13

At 8 a.m. Dr. Jewett emails: "We discussed your case yesterday and recommended surgery including removal of the involved piece of rib. We communicated that opinion to Dr. X." I sit by the telephone, but no one from Dr. X's office bothers to call. At mid-afternoon I call Dr. X's office. No one returns my message. Do you know how it feels to be abandoned by your doctor after he's let you know you're likely a stage IV cancer? You expect the medics to rush to lend you a hand and instead you meet a deep and hurtful silence. Everyone has had the frustrating experience of dealing with an indifferent bureaucracy, but when the stakes are your very life, the non-response is traumatic. I've encountered several of the lower-echelon workers at PMH, the receptionists and administrative assistants, and some of them call to mind the powerful bunglers in Franz Kafka's novel *The Trial*. We take such encounters to be unique to our modern age. But there is a Midrash that tells of a sinful King David begging God to deal with him directly and not give him into the hands of the lower-level seraphim and cherubim. As King David notes, these assistants are cruel. In Kafka's world, they are maddeningly disorganized and thoughtless.

Do all government-sponsored institutions, regardless of the political system, breed indifference? In the mid-1980s I spent some time lecturing in Beijing. In the slovenly run department stores the salespeople took a perverse delight in ignoring you, and when they did go to retrieve the socks you asked for (everything was behind counters under lock and key) they did so grudgingly. At the airport, the baggage handlers and ticket agents seemed indifferent to departure times. In all the government agencies one noted a smouldering resentment.

As the day wears on and the telephone remains silent, I shrink; I feel powerless; I feel small and inconsequential.

I think of the phrase "fall through the cracks."

Like a grain of rice on a splintered table, I have fallen through the cracks.

I am ashamed to admit that I call Dr. X's office five more times that day and leave more messages, but what else is there to do?

I could have saved my breath.

I will never hear from Dr. X again.

Wednesday, April 14

Over breakfast, Marie and I discuss my situation. We decide it would be in my best interest to fax Dr. Jewett a request that he take over my case, along with all my records. He has proven to be a considerate man who is willing to communicate with me. Sid, my GP, has my records, so this morning Marie and I drove to his office to ask Nellie, Sid's receptionist, to fax my request, along with my records, to Dr. Jewett. Later, Sid phones and advises strongly against the move. His reason is twofold. First, it will slow down the process, as he believes that sooner or later Dr. X will come through. Second, it will antagonize the doctors, who work together in the same department at PMH. Reluctantly I heed his advice, but I ask myself what sort of health-care system we have devised for ourselves. I can walk into four different clothing stores to check out the neckties, but when it comes to my all-important health my choices are more limited. One can see why the Americans are skittish about adopting our system: while it does relieve the patient of the worry of cost—a tremendous burden to a significant portion of the population—it also restricts freedom of choice, a value that Americans hold dear.

Thursday, April 15

All along I have had an ace in my hand without knowing it. My cousin Ferne Sherkin is married to Dr. Jack Langer, a highly respected pediatric surgeon at Toronto's Sick Kids' Hospital. For days, Marie has been urging me to get in touch with Jack and I have resisted, partly because of pride (I like to believe that I can manage on my own), and partly because I doubt that a pediatric surgeon would have any influence with the urological surgeons at PMH. But I am at my wit's end in thinking of ways to break through the system and get myself the surgery I need. I email cousin Ferne who immediately sends me Jack's cellphone number. I leave him a message at 10 a.m. and at 10:30 he returns my call. I tell him the details of my case and the quagmire I find myself in. Jack tells me that he knows Michael Jewett both personally and professionally and describes him as "very experienced and also a wonderful person." I cannot believe my luck. Jack tells me he will get back and one hour later he phones to tell me that he has spoken with Michael Jewett. "I think you can expect things to move more quickly now," Jack says. Then cautiously, "I guess you know there's a rib involved." I tell Jack that I'm aware of that.

"I wasn't sure you knew," he says. "Anyway," Jack continues, "Jewett's not convinced the bone tumour is malignant."

I savour this small ray of hope.

Jack asks me if I have told my parents about my condition and I tell him that I haven't. I explain to him that I do not want to burden my parents, who are in their eighties, with distressing news, but the real reason I haven't told them is our conflicted relationship. I'm not sure that contending with them won't add to my stress.

"You should tell them," Jack advises. "If they know they can be supportive. You don't want to be alone with this."

Jack's comments have me thinking about the pros and cons of disclosure. In the case of my parents, I sense they already know something is up when they hear my voice or Marie's. At this point, it would be easier to tell them than to continue hiding the truth. Covering up proves to be enervating, and appears to be a poor strategy after all. If I'd not been so tight-lipped about my disease, Jack Langer would have known about my condition weeks ago and I wouldn't have had to needlessly suffer. Are you not more likely to receive the help you need by standing on a rooftop and shouting "Fire!" at the top of your lungs than by hiding yourself in a room and waiting to hear from unresponsive doctors?

8

Later in the day, at 6:43 p.m., to be precise, I receive an email from Dr. Jewett confirming that he has spoken with Jack Langer. He tells me that Dr. X is going on holiday and that either he or "our partner and kidney cancer expert Dr. Tony Finelli" will be operating on me. He tells me that he has put in a request for thoracic surgery to see me, as we may need their help with the operation. This is the first time I have heard the term "thoracic surgery." After the call, I Google it and discover it is surgery involving the chest cavity. I am already in a state of heightened anxiety and worry that there are metastatic spots on my lungs that I have not been told about. I email Jack Langer asking why the need for a thoracic surgeon: and he lets me know that a thoracic surgeon is needed to remove the affected rib. I am learning as I go along.

Friday, April 16

I slept better last night. I feel grateful to Jack Langer, for I am no longer a grain of rice that has slipped through the cracks. In the USA, money can buy you the best insurance and speedy, good-quality health care. This system seems to work for the upper stratum of the population, though it is not a solution for those who are poor. (I am not a health-care expert, but I wonder whether we in Canada need a system that allows some private coverage for those who can afford it, if only to take pressure off the government-assisted hospitals.)

At PMH, money would not have helped me, unless the money had also brought connections or notoriety. If you read the cancer memoirs by celebrities in this country (it would be unseemly of me to mention names) you will find that they do not experience wait time. Neither do politicians. In Canada, recognition replaces money. Those who are known are on the fast track to care.

As Jack promised, things are beginning to move. Around noon I receive a call from Dr. X's office, informing me that Dr. X will be away for some time and that my case is being transferred to Dr. Tony Finelli. I will hear from Finelli's office.

Three hours later a different woman from Dr. X's office calls to inform me that a surgery date with Dr. X has been set for late May. When I tell her that my case has been transferred to Dr. Finelli and that someone from her office has already phoned to tell me so, she asks, "Are you sure?"

A harmless mix-up? I find it unsettling. If they cannot get this right, I say to myself, then what assurance do I have when it comes time to operate they will not remove my healthy right kidney and leave the cancerous left one intact?

I receive one final call this afternoon from PMH. It is Dr. X's nurse, the one who commiserated with Marie. I have not heard from her since the day I called to enquire about my bone scan. She wants me to know that she and her team will do everything they can to make my transition to Dr. Finelli's office as smooth and as timely as possible. I thank her but do not believe her. Not because she is a liar, but because she has no control over this flawed and plodding bureaucracy. She tells me what I already suspect: that Dr. Jewett had been to the clinic to enquire about my case. (Wanting to know, I assume, why this grain of rice had fallen through the cracks.)

Monday, April 19

I do not hear from Dr. Finelli's office in the morning. In the afternoon, I get through to Massy, Dr. Finelli's assistant, who will prove to be a bright and efficient ally in my quest for treatment. Massy tells me that she knows of the transfer but has received no paperwork from Dr. X's office, and until she receives that paperwork nothing can be done. Why am I not surprised?

Tuesday, April 20

I phone Massy in the morning but can't get through. I phone again in the afternoon. ("The man suffering from a character-ized sickness is not entitled to complain: he has an occupa-tion.") She has at last received the paperwork. Dr. Finelli can see me for a consult on May 6: that's nearly two and a half long, agonizing weeks from today. At that time he will discuss a surgery date, which will likely be sometime in early July. This is outrageous. If I am operated upon in early July it will mean

I'll have waited three and a half months from the time Sid felt the tumour. I tell Massy my story and plead for an earlier consult date. She puts me on hold and comes back with a consult date of April 29. She will see what she can do about an earlier surgery date but cannot, at this time, commit.

That evening I receive a phone call from Sid, my family doctor. He has kept in contact with me and knows that I am still waiting for a surgery date. His voice becomes emotional as he lets me know that he's left messages with Dr. X's office and that they have not even had the courtesy to return his calls. He apologizes for not being able to get me the care I need and wonders aloud whether the entire health-care system should be dismantled and rebuilt, from the foundation up. I'm touched by Sid's phone call, by his humanity. I tell him about Jack Langer and how things have started to move along.

I have been emailing Jack, apprising him of the situation, expressing frustration with the delay in getting surgery, and he has been helping me to focus on the big picture.

"They may be postponing some other less urgent cases to get your operation done, so it probably takes some arranging," Jack informs me.

I go into more details about the Kafkaesque hospital bureaucracy I've encountered.

"This is one of the downsides of our health-care system," Jack says, "and those of us who are in the delivery side are extremely frustrated as well with the limitations on O.R. time, clinic space, etcetera, that make it so challenging to provide timely, top-quality care. However, in the big picture you'll be getting the best care possible from world-class experts, and ultimately that's what's most important."

Part Two

Wednesday, April 21

I have not been able to write much poetry. It is not so much the lack of time as the ongoing angst that inhibits creativity. This adds to my despair because for me the writing, the engagement with language, is what has gotten me through times of trouble. I have been able to read, though, and am immersed in the memoir *Life Work* by the American poet Donald Hall; it is a paean to joyful labour interrupted by an episode of cancer that threatened Hall's life. Hall's models for meaningful work are (a) his farmer grandparents who worked the soil of Connecticut, (b) Henry Moore, the prolific sculptor, and (c) Sigmund Freud, the father of psychoanalysis and a fellow cancer patient.

Freud loved work. At the height of his career in Vienna, he kept a strict routine: into bed at one in the morning, rise at seven, conduct analysis with patients from eight to twelve. He'd lunch with his family at one, and then take a walk to buy his much-loved cigars. At three he began another series of appointments, and oftentimes saw patients until nine at night. After supper he'd walk to a café with his wife then return home to read, write, and edit. On Saturdays he lectured from five to seven and then played cards with friends. Sundays, he answered letters.

When Freud grew old he had to deal with two catastrophes: jaw cancer and the rise of Hitler. At the eleventh hour he escaped Vienna for England, but from his cancer there was no escape. He came to England with a jaw prosthesis, which made it possible for him to eat and talk, though it caused him considerable pain.

Work, Freud believed, is an effective technique to fend off suffering, and he considered some forms of work especially effective, "such as an artist's joy in creating." But he conceded that even the creative process is not full proof in combatting unhappiness. In his late masterwork, *Civilization and Its Discontents*, he acknowledges that to those who possess "special dispositions and gifts this method cannot give complete protection from suffering. It creates no impenetrable armour against the arrows of misfortune ..." Referring to his own painful and debilitating experience with cancer, Freud notes that work's restorative power "habitually fails when the source of the suffering is a person's own body."

I am not suffering physical pain, yet, but the psychic turmoil has worried away my muse. I wait for the radiant immediacy of words to return, for the healing grace of language.

8

Marie's father had told us, as we walked the corridor of the North York General Hospital, that he did not view his illness as a punishment. Can I say the same? I think my father-in-law was admirable and atypical. I believe that most people with a disease carry some punitive notions around it.

How do I think about my cancer? Disbelief was my initial reaction. I was astonished that my body—without providing me with the least inkling of what it was up to—nurtured a tumour measuring fifteen centimetres. The average kidney measures twelve to thirteen centimetres. This means that my kidney tumour overshadows my kidney. I picture this tumour as my kidney's nefarious double, my Bizarro World kidney, if you will. From what I have read about the development of renal tumours, I estimate that my cancerous mass began its growth ten years ago. That means a decade of insidious, malignant development, without a single symptom, without a single sign. The disconnect between my body and myself is haunting and leaves me with a sense of awe regarding my cancer. I marvel at its craftiness, its ability to sneak up on me and kill me without rustling a leaf or shaking a branch. One has to fear and admire such a resourceful enemy.

Overriding that sense of admiration is my enormous disappointment. How could my body, which I have cared for so lovingly by avoiding abuse and overindulgence, let me down? How could it have been fooled into producing this cancer that Samson-like, threatens to tear down the entire edifice?

My traitorous body, betraying the trust I have invested in it.

My defective body, unable to recognize a healthy, normal cell from one that carries death.

My dumb, silent body.

Thursday, April 22

What role does the imagination play when we think about illness?

The first book I read on the subject of disease was Susan Sontag's elegant classic *Illness as Metaphor*. I read the book when it first appeared in 1978 and now that I am a resident in Sontag's "kingdom of the sick," I decide to read it again.

Given her own disturbing cancer experience, Sontag's restraint and objectivity toward her subject are remarkable. She gives not the slightest hint of the panic she must have felt when at age forty-two she was diagnosed with advanced-stage breast cancer. Her goal in writing such an analytical book was utilitarian. As she explained ten years after *Illness as Metaphor* was published: "I didn't think it would be useful—and I wanted to be useful—to tell yet one more story in the first person of how someone learned that he or she had cancer, wept, struggled, was comforted, suffered, took courage … though mine was also that story."

Turning her penetrating gaze on illness imagery in literature and film, Sontag exposes some unpleasant and unacknowledged truths. She tells us that our views on illness are imbued with shame, fear, and self-vilification.

We disparage the seriously sick. Worse, the sick disparage themselves. Sontag intended her study as an antidote to the poisonous perceptions we hold about disease because, she believed, those perceptions "deform the experience of having cancer." She hoped that her sober analysis might rid the patient of fearful metaphors (for instance, the sci-fi scenario in which the patient imagines him- or herself invaded by mutant or alien cells) and the awful self-negation that a dire diagnosis often triggers. Once liberated from those metaphoric trappings and critical pitfalls, the patient would make the best choices for treatment.

While I admire Sontag's attempt to strip cancer of its harmful associations, and while I agree with her that it is more helpful to think of illness as biological mishap than as the result of personality defect, I question her idea that "the most truthful way of regarding illness—and the healthiest way of being ill—is one most purified of, most resistant to, metaphoric thinking." In the grip of my cancer experience—an experience that forces the imagination to work overtime—I wonder if that is possible, or even wise.

A few paragraphs earlier I credited my cancer with the "ability to sneak up on me and kill me without rustling a leaf or shaking a branch." That metaphor came to me soon after I was diagnosed. The truth is, once you hear the news of your illness, the metaphoric thinking begins. It rarely lets up.

I find it impossible to avoid thinking about my disease in metaphors, just as I found it impossible, at first, to avoid self-blame. I worried that I grew this tumour because I hadn't eaten properly or had drunk water that was unfiltered. Perhaps my cancer was the result of those asbestos tiles I'd removed from the basement ceiling of our house soon after we moved in. Maybe it was the result of keeping my feelings bottled up, of leading a life of quiet desperation.

You can really work yourself over once you have a serious illness. For the most part I am able to limit the amount of self-blame by reminding myself that science has yet to unlock the biochemical links to cancer. At present, most forms of the disease are viewed as the result of random, spontaneous mutations. Bad luck. But I cannot stop the flow of imagery, and my intuition suggests that it would be unhealthy to repress the figurative reimagining of my illness. I know from my years of reading and composing poetry that image-making is a vital dialogue with the self.

Giving my imagination free rein, I discover allies in the other books I am reading. Shortly after he was diagnosed with advanced prostate cancer, Anatole Broyard, the one-time literary critic for *The New York Times*, wrote, "the sick man sees everything as metaphor." He viewed this as a plus. In his book, *Intoxicated by My Illness*, Broyard criticized Sontag for "being too hard on metaphor." As he says, "metaphors may be as necessary to illness as they are to literature.... At the very least, they are a relief from medical terminology.... [O]nly metaphor can express the bafflement, the panic combined with beatitude of the threatened person." Broyard wrote his book as he was dying. Illness books that are written while the angel of death hovers near are exceptionally rich in metaphor. Novelist Harold Brodkey, dying of AIDS, described himself as "a small bird nervous in the shadow, a bag of tainted blood ..." It's as if figurative language were acting as a type of palliative.

Poet John Keats praised "the truth of the Imagination," and my cancer experience has me thinking that such truth originates in our very cells. Reading Dr. Siddhartha Mukherjee's *The Emperor of All Maladies*, I am startled to realize that envisioning my cancer as an ill-intentioned double, a malignant disguised version of myself, is in keeping with recent scientific assessments. For Mukherjee, cancer is "a parallel species ... more adapted to survival than we are." He deems it "our desperate, malevolent, contemporary doppelganger." His amazement rests on one undeniable fact: "Cancer cells can grow faster, adapt better. They are more perfect versions of ourselves." Such figurative language captures the awe, the astonishment of having cancer. I prefer it to the cold, clinical terminology of the CT scan report I was handed with my diagnosis.

I often envision my tumour as a fetus getting larger and larger, myself pregnant with approaching death. My doctors have speculated that the cancer has metastasized, and I picture the malignant cells coursing through my blood as spy ships sent out from Tumour Central, looking for other organs to invade. I know that none of these imaginings are unique or out of the ordinary. Once you read a number of illness memoirs, you realize that being sick can render your imagination quotidian; it's a levelling experience that binds you to suffering humanity. Of course, if you're a talented writer, à la Brodkey, you can convey your experience in language that is fresh and startling. Moreover, *pace* Sontag, my own metaphoric thinking hasn't deterred me from seeking the best treatment. On the contrary, the terror of my imaginings keeps me phoning for earlier appointments, quicker results.

Despite my efforts to get a date for surgery, I am forced to wait. I find reading is the best way to deal with this wait time. After I complete my rereading of *Illness as Metaphor*, I dip into Sontag's newly published journals, edited by her son, David Rieff. I also read the harrowing memoir *Swimming in a Sea of Death*, which Rieff wrote about his mother's third, and final, battle with cancer. What I hadn't known when I read Sontag's *Illness as Metaphor* was that it had been written, in Rieff's words, "long after her treatments had ended and all seemed to be well," when she could look back on her frightening experience with some degree of equanimity. In the mid-1970s,

Sontag had been diagnosed with stage IV metastatic breast cancer (the disease had spread to seventeen of her lymph nodes), and doctors at New York's Sloan Kettering Cancer Center held out little hope. Driven by a strong will to survive, Sontag did her own research and found a doctor in Paris who was willing to administer a more aggressive, experimental chemotherapy regime; this likely saved her life. But Rieff discloses that when his mother was first diagnosed, she engaged in the same sort of punishing emotions and metaphoric thinking that she later warned others against. For instance, upon learning of her illness, she played the self-blame game. As an intellectual, she had flirted with the highly suspect Reichian theory, which held that blocked desires—especially sexual desires—cause cancer. "I'm responsible for my cancer," she wrote in one of her journals. "I lived as a coward, repressing my desire, my rage." And when she began chemotherapy, she indulged in extreme forms of metaphoric thinking: "I feel like the Vietnam War," she wrote. "My body is invasive, colonizing. They're using chemical weapons on me." Given her inquisitive and polemical nature, at some point after her illness Sontag began to question what she had thought and felt about having cancer. The skeptical brilliance of *Illness as Metaphor* speaks of one who's come through and wishes to dispel the defeatist, punitive notions of cancer so that those who follow may be less burdened. A noble project. But Rieff argues, convincingly, that it was not Sontag's analytical powers so much as her obstinate attachment to living (what he calls "my mother's steely resolve") that guided her choice of aggressive therapies and prolonged her life.

When I finish reading Rieff's memoir I realize that the time Sontag waited to write her classic book allowed her to distance herself from an experience she found excruciatingly painful. It permitted her to think critically about our social and historical attitudes toward cancer. But her distancing also cut her off from the immediacy of the sickness experience and led her to limit our imaginings, unaware that our metaphors are the deepest expressions we have, and that by voicing them we tap a source of inner strength.

8

Do thoughts and emotions contribute to illness? Can they help us get better? Shortly after Marie was diagnosed with breast cancer, we enrolled in the Healing Journey, a course devised and run by Alastair Cunningham of PMH. Cunningham, a survivor of stage III colon cancer, offers a "spiritual" approach to the treatment of cancer. Marie and I would alleviate our stress by playing Alastair's relaxation tape, which asks you to clench a specific part of your body and then relax. *Clench your jaw; hold it; let go; tighten your stomach muscles; count to ten; let go.* At the end of the tape Alastair asks you to picture yourself in a time and place where you feel at peace. I always choose my childhood at the summer cottage. I have rowed out to the point, the spot beyond the bay that is known for good fishing. I have my rod, my stringer, my takeout container filled with thick dew worms weaving through black and golden moss. In case the worms don't do the trick, I have a Styrofoam container filled with cold water in which leeches stretch like black elastic bands. I have a small red toolbox with extra tackle: hooks, bobs, sinkers, a spare reel. I have a transistor radio, but I use it sparingly. I prefer the silence, broken now and then by the cry of gulls. I contemplate the grim-mouthed bass, moving through the frigid depths, circling my bait. I am always alone in my imagined moment of peace, far from family and neighbours. The sky is clear and the breeze off the lake, invigorating. Is this why I love to write? The blank page is the unruffled surface of the lake. I plumb the depths, hoping for a strike.

During one of his sessions, Alastair asks us to picture our cancer cells as black-hatted meanies. We are asked to imagine our chemotherapy drugs, or our radiation, or our positive feelings, as white-hatted sheriffs who have come to drive the black-hats out of town. There is nothing wrong in marshalling positive forces, but I have reservations about this particular use of metaphor as a healing technique. It has the potential to set the patient up to be a loser: I am dying because I did not believe strongly enough in the power of my sheriff. I am dying because I allowed meanies to overrun the town.

What exactly are the connections between the body's health and the workings of the imagination? Science has yet to understand them. One thing we do know: you can think positively and still succumb to a deadly form of cancer, or you can think the darkest thoughts and survive. Knowing this, I am free to let my mind wonder without worrying that my catastrophic fantasies will assist my cancer cells.

8

One day, while surfing the Internet, I find an article titled "The Therapeutic Psychopoetics of Cancer Metaphors," by Ulrich Teucher, a professor of psychology at the University of Saskatchewan. I am drawn to the term "psychopoetics." Teucher contends that in a crisis "metaphor functions primarily to stabilize our selves in uncertainty and change and to distance us from fearful chaos." It's hardly surprising then that cancer discourse teems with metaphors, since, as Teucher rightly observes "Cancer presents one of the most terrifying epitomes of the unknown."

To gather data on what images we associate with cancer, Teucher asked participants—a mix of cancer patients and persons without cancer—to complete a detailed questionnaire. The cancer patients were encouraged to write a brief narrative. He grouped the responses into five basic sets of metaphors, or "clusters," as he calls them.

1. **Invasion:** Here we have words like "attack," "opponent," "battle." Martial metaphors are the most common to

cancer: hospitals ask us to donate so that we can "beat cancer in our lifetime." Governments declare "a war against cancer." Newspapers tell us that a celebrity "succumbed after a long battle with cancer."

2. **Intrusion:** These are images of a less belligerent nature such as "unwelcome intruder" and "the thief that steals time."

3. **Oppressive Surroundings:** Patients say that they are under a "dark cloud" or within a "scary cave."

4. **Growth Inside:** Patients report "being eaten from the inside out," overtaken by a "parasite," or enduring a "demonic pregnancy."

5. **Obstacles:** Patients feel as though they have come up against a "stone wall" or a "hard stroke of fate."

Teucher's article was published in 2003. I notice that cancer metaphors have morphed over time as more is learned of the disease's biological genesis. If Teucher ran his survey today, he'd likely find a number of patients picturing their cancer as a malicious double, thriving among their unsuspecting organs.

Friday, April 23

I am seeing Dr. Finelli in six days and have not heard from Massy, his receptionist, regarding an earlier date for my operation. She mentioned early July, but let's say she can pull off a miracle and get me in one month earlier. That would mean I will have waited ten weeks since the tumour was discovered. Is that acceptable? The government of Ontario maintains a website devoted to recording wait times for different types of surgeries. For genitourinary cancers (kidney, bladder, penile, prostate, testicular, urethral, and ureter) the average provincial wait time, I discover, is fifty-seven days, or close to two months. For PMH, I see that the average is eighty-five days, or close to three months. There is a link that lets me know where I can find the shortest wait time for this type of surgery: it is

Woodstock General Hospital. Twenty-three days. If I have the surgery at PMH in early July, when Massy first suggested, I will have waited three and a half months, 105 days. (Remember, 85 days is only the average.) Early June will give me eighty-five days, or the average. And while I wait, I know full well that the cancer could be spreading to other bones and organs.

My brother urges me to call his friend's uncle, an oncologist at the Mayo Clinic, who provides me with the name of their top kidney cancer surgeon. I call the office of Dr. Bradley C. Leibovich, and his cheerful assistant listens attentively to the details of my case and takes down all the pertinent information. I do not feel rushed. Unlike the personnel one often speaks to at PMH, Dr. Leibovich's assistant is not harried. She suggests I fax all the information and test results to her office. She assures me that if I commit to having the surgery the operation will be done in three to four weeks. She tells me the operation will cost a minimum of $30,000 US dollars but that other charges may be levied for drugs and tests. She asks whether I want Dr. Leibovich to call me later in the afternoon to discuss my case over the phone. I find the mere thought of a surgeon willing to speak with me over the phone a comfort, and realize that *our* health-care system exacerbates the aloneness that the cancer patient already feels. The seriously ill patient craves to connect with his healers, but such a connection is difficult within an overtaxed system. The patient is left feeling as though his potential healers are indifferent to his plight.

Given my financial situation, I quickly determine that the Mayo's cost for surgery is prohibitive. I thank Dr. Leibovich's assistant for her time and decide that when I meet Dr. Finelli I will plead for an earlier surgery date.

8

Who is Dr. Antonio Finelli? A graduate of the University of Toronto, he completed a fellowship at the Cleveland Clinic and is expert at laparoscopic surgery. Dr. Finelli is interested primarily in prostate and renal cancers. I email Dr. Steven Gallinger, asking his opinion of Dr. Finelli and he emails me back saying he has heard that he is an excellent surgeon and assures me that I will be "in good hands." When I check the website RateMDs.com, I see that Dr. Finelli is rated five out of five, based on nineteen reviews. "AMAZING" is the word used by three respondents, all using capital letters. Another says he "rocks." The general consensus is that he is caring, diligent, and responsive. ("Answers emails!" one entrant exults.) This is encouraging. I really need someone who is AMAZING to conquer my cancer.

Thursday, April 29

Does one ever wait calmly in the reception area of a cancer clinic? I never have. My nervousness makes it difficult for me to focus on the *New Yorker* magazine I have brought with me. My name is called and Marie and I are led to the examination room. Soon after, Dr. Tony Finelli passes by. I recognize him from the photo on the PMH website: Mediterranean complexion, dark eyes, wavy black hair. He is wearing a purple shirt and black trousers. Stylish. Not everyone can successfully wear a purple shirt. To do so requires confidence. Finelli, I am relieved to note, has flair. I choose to think of the colourful shirt and black trousers as clothes a toreador might wear. Here is someone, I imagine, who can slay the rampaging bull.

How rational is the relationship that the patient has with his doctor? The patient is looking for someone to conquer his illness. The patient is looking for someone who understands his terror, his hopes, his confusion and disappointments. How reasonable is all this to ask of anyone?

And what about the doctor? What are his goals, besides healing? Has he been taught to keep a professional distance between himself and the patient? What does such distancing cost, in psychological terms? Wouldn't it be easier if the doctor welcomed the human dimensions of the patient?

8

Dr. Finelli passes our room a second time and stops.

"Mr. and Mrs. Sherman?"

"Yes."

"I'll be with you in a minute. I have one follow-up to see which will take a minute or two."

Dr. Finelli acknowledges us. He is considerate. He returns with four young medical students in tow and asks if I mind their sitting in. The students are in white lab coats and because each possesses the same flat expression, I find them indistinguishable. This is their field trip to the Land of Cancer and I tell Finelli that I do not mind their being present. I am in the education field myself. And I have accepted that I am now a specimen, to be observed, to be discussed.

Finelli begins in a surprising way: he acknowledges my recent struggles by telling the students that navigating our health-care system can be frustrating, difficult. He tells them how my general practitioner discovered my tumour, and praises the hands of Dr. Sidney Nusinowich. He goes over the ultrasound and CT scan results in some detail, addressing the students but also turning to look me in the eye to remind me that though he is using me as a teaching specimen, he still regards me as a human being. He then informs his students that cancer cells from the primary tumour are "likely" in my blood stream, and that my bone lesion is "most likely" the result of metastasis. He surprises me a second time by proclaiming to the students that my prognosis is good. How in God's name, I wonder, can my prognosis be good? The answer seems to rest upon Sutent and its related drugs. Oncologists and pharmaceutical companies call them "wonder drugs" because they have the power to shrink and control metastatic tumours. In some exceptional cases they can fully eliminate cancer cells in the body.

Finelli describes, briefly, the two surgeries I will have: one to excise my left kidney, the other to remove a segment of my ninth posterior rib. He tells the students that early on there was a suggestion from the Tumour Board to use Sutent before surgery in an attempt to reduce the size of the tumour. This, he says, is still an option.

This is news to me. "I thought the Tumour Board had discounted that option and advised surgery," I pipe up.

Finelli explains that he and the oncologist Dr. Jennifer Knox are carrying out a clinical trial to determine the outcomes of those who take preoperative drugs. I can be part of that trial if I choose. The drugs, he explains, can possibly shrink the primary tumour but will have little effect on the rib lesion. I'm not sure what the best course of action is, but because this news has been sprung on me, I feel justified in asking Dr. Finelli, in front of his students, what he would do if he were in my shoes.

I have caught him off guard. "Sheesh," he says. He takes a moment to rebound and says, "Given that I am a surgeon, I would opt for the surgery first."

Fair enough.

Finelli dismisses his students. He informs me that my surgery date will be Wednesday, May 26. That is more than three weeks from today; two and a half months since Sid found the tumour. I ask if he can operate sooner, but due to the backlog of waiting patients, May 26 is the very best he can do. He tells me that scheduling has already put me ahead of some other patients to compensate for the bureaucratic bumbling. He cannot do better.

"In the three and a half weeks that we wait for surgery, my cancer could spread further," I remind Dr. Finelli.

"That is correct," he concedes.

He advises me not to think too much about the surgery. He asks me to try and relax and save my energy for the operation.

"You don't seem tired," he says. "A tumour as big as yours consumes large quantities of blood. You're likely anemic. Many patients complain of tiredness."

I tell him that I ran five kilometres this morning.

"The fact that you feel good is a positive sign," he says. "Don't focus on the size of the tumour. Don't let it get you down. I once had a female patient whose kidney tumour extended from her abdomen down to her groin. It was huge! Incredibly, there was no metastasis."

"She was one lucky lady," I reply.

Dr. Finelli then asks me if I've ever had surgery and I tell him that I never have.

"I'm going to be straight with you," he says. "This is going to be a major hit. A double surgery. I will remove the kidney, then we will turn you over and the thoracic surgeon will remove a segment of your rib. We will try to control the pain, but you will be hurting afterwards."

I appreciate his directness. It frees me from illusion. I especially like the word "hit." You want a doctor who will use expressive language. It shows style, independence of mind.

Like donning a purple shirt.

Wednesday, May 5

7:45 a.m. I am at PMH for my pre-op. The nurses are attentive, considerate, and informative. They take my blood pressure, ask about allergies, weigh and measure me. They let me know that I will have pain after my surgery. There will be attempts to control it: a pain management team will come around and ask me to rank my pain on a scale of one to ten. They can then prescribe medication. The pre-op nurses are upfront about letting me know that nothing will take the pain down to a grade of zero.

I am asked to elect either a morphine pump or a pre-operative epidural to get me over the hump of post-surgical pain. I choose the epidural, based on the experience of my friend David Redgrave. Since my diagnosis, David, the survivor of four separate cancers, has served as my model and coach. He is a member of the poetry workshop I conduct each Monday evening. British-born and with a degree in economics, David served as an advisor to several of Ontario's finance ministers dating back to the government of John Robarts. When David was in his mid-thirties he developed an aggressive melanoma that he miraculously survived. "Everything after that," he says, "has been gravy." In his early sixties he was diagnosed with colon cancer and had part of his intestines removed. Two months later, during his recovery from the colon cancer, an ultrasound revealed a tumour on his kidney. Doctors couldn't tell whether it was a spread from the colon cancer or a cancer of the kidney. A biopsy of the growth revealed the latter. David had his third separate cancer. Then, two years ago, as we walked to our cars after a poetry session, David nonchalantly informed me that he'd recently been diagnosed with prostate cancer. A four-bagger. I drove him to a few of his radiation treatments. When I told him about my kidney cancer he lifted his jersey to show off the sickle-shaped scar along his flank. When I asked about the pain treatment option, David advised an epidural. "It's a no-brainer," he said. Other advice? "After your surgery, shave and dress every day. Don't appear slovenly. Don't let yourself go. And don't complain to the doctors. Doctors hate a whiner." David is eighty. He plays a fine stride piano. He likes Jelly Roll Morton. He likes the poetry of Wallace Stevens. He still has all his hair and all his marbles.

Witty and understated, David gives the impression of having walked through his cancers. Of course, he hasn't. He's careful to remind me that his wife, Dorith, has been beside him through every medical trial—some of which he calls "cliffhangers."

"Dorith was the one who chased the system for additional care whenever I got too stoical or was ready to give up," David informs me. "She was my formidable reason for thinking and acting 'survival.'" He wonders aloud whether he'd survived his cancers had he been living alone. "There's a psychic side to fighting sickness," he observes, "in which husbands and wives are more than just bystanders."

Are there statistics to prove David's observation that close relationships assist in survival? I think of the help I gave Marie when she was going through her breast cancer treatment. I think of the help she is giving me and find it alarming to imagine living alone with my fears and frustrations. Whether you survive or die, isn't it best to hear a calming voice, to feel a comforting hand in yours?

Thursday, May 13

3 p.m. Marie and I wait in the examination room at the thoracic clinic. Dr. Y, my designated surgeon, is now forty-five minutes late for our appointment. I am staring at the puke-beige walls, at the white porcelain sink: who ever thought that this sparse, lab-like ambience would encourage a patient? I wonder whether the design owes itself to the idea of asepsis, the avoidance of contagion. Once upon a time the patient's health was protected by the sterility of the hospital, but, as Anatole Broyard observed, "the sterility went too far. It sterilized the doctor's thinking. It sterilized the patient's entire experience in the hospital. It sterilized our very notion of illness to the point where we can't bring our soiled thoughts to bear on it. But the sick man needs the contagion of life."

"Death," Broyard rightly notes, "is the ultimate sterility." I agree with Broyard and think that the patient, in a hospital setting, should be reminded of life. There ought to be paintings and drawings on the walls, sculpture on the little desk where patient and doctor discuss their strategies to defeat disease.

There ought to be some calming classical music piped into the room to alleviate the abysmal silence that envelopes the anxious patient and his caregiver.

Broyard has a more radical idea; he suggests that the examination room be modelled after a mini-theatre. It's an idea worth considering. To the patient, a serious illness is certainly life's central drama. The modern examination room diminishes the experience, making illness a paltry event.

8

Dr. Y arrives and excuses herself for being late. She is clearly flustered and begins by telling us she spent the morning as a witness at a malpractice trial, testifying on behalf of a colleague. This has put her behind in her schedule. She spends several minutes recounting what her fellow doctor did wrong and explaining to us that mistakes can happen. Doctors, she informs us, are fallible. We nod and say that we are sure that mistakes can happen. It does not seem to occur to Dr. Y that I am not here to listen to the trials and tribulations of thoracic surgeons. I have metastatic kidney cancer and am anxious to hear how Dr. Y is going to deal with my malignant rib. On the other hand, her venting makes her human in my eyes.

Is Dr. Y a good surgeon? My operation is in two weeks and I do not have time to investigate or shop around. One thing for certain is that she is incapable of putting her moment in court behind her, as it seems to have rattled her. When she examines me she places her hand on my lower back and begins to count up from my bottom rib to the ninth, where she presses down attempting to feel the tumour. She repeats this count twice, telling us that it is quite possible to cut into the wrong rib. This I take to be a legal disclaimer. I tell Dr. Y that I find it incredible, with modern imaging techniques, that a surgeon could remove the wrong rib.

"Oh, it does happen," Dr. Y assures me.

Marie and I tell her we're confident she'll find the ninth rib and get the tumour out. We find ourselves in the odd position of having to reassure the doctor. Shouldn't it be the doctor who reassures us? Later, at the Hope Street Café, we laugh about our meeting with Dr. Y, but it is dark laughter. You put your anesthetized self in the hands of a surgeon, a person about whom you know very little. What if it turns out that she is incompetent, or addicted to drugs? You are out cold on the operating table, and there's the unknown surgeon stooping over you with her scalpel, checking the CT scan, and feeling for the right rib before making her incision. Did she get enough sleep the night before? Did she have an argument with her spouse? Does she have arthritis? Is there anything at all distracting her from the job at hand?

Saturday, May 15

Now that I have a firm date for my operation I find that my anxiety drops a notch. I am able to write poems again.

It rained the day we had our appointment with Dr. Y, so I had brought with me my five-dollar New York umbrella. I call it that because as we were about to leave the MoMA last year during our trip to New York City it began to pour. A number of umbrella hawkers sprouted up on 53rd Street in front of the main entrance to the museum. Spontaneous American capitalism. The umbrella conjures memories of that trip. We were visiting our son, Adam. The photo studio where he works is in the Meatpacking District in a building that overlooks the Hudson. When Sully Sullenberger landed his damaged plane on the river, in what is now known as the Miracle on the Hudson, Adam snapped photos from the window of his studio. On the day we saw Dr. Y, the rain brought out my umbrella as well as recollections of Manhattan, and that led to the thought—astonishing how the mind weaves its way to where it needs to go—that I too was in need of a miracle.

Umbrella

It smells of the molten metropolis,
of asphalt and tar

and folds into the palm of my hand
compact as a bat, silent, aware

ready to open like a judicial robe
against the rage of unexpected weather.

Thin as my skin and like my skin
it remembers downpour, drizzle,

drops that build slowly as tears (words
grow stale but tears are always fresh).

Dark canopy
to shield against sky's darkness.

I continue to be amazed by the life-sustaining, life-enhancing, and unpredictable nature of poetry—its random arrival—and by its ability to convey the mystery of one's inner life. What else do I possess, other than poetry, to confront the "rage of unexpected weather"?

What are the secret sources of a poem? Behind that memory of the deluge outside of the MoMA, there stands a doctor informing me that I am seriously ill. No doctor is mentioned in the poem, but he's there, whispering between the lines. Who would guess that the poem's tone of urgency is a response to his diagnosis? If I want, I can interpret the poem's figurative language in the light of my illness. The images speak to my vulnerability ("thin as my skin"), to my sorrow ("drops that build slowly as tears"), and to my wish for protection ("dark canopy"). None of this actually *explains* the poem, but the images hint at what I take to be the emotional forces behind its conception. What is important for me is that I was able, while composing the poem, to transcend my dread and suffering.

And the reader is fortified too, since when you read a poem you experience a metamorphosis—you become the poet.

Monday, May 17

Have I done enough for myself? It will be almost two and a half months from the time Sid felt my tumour to the day of my operation. What more could I have done? As I sit and read, or work now and then on my poems, I wonder whether the cancer is spreading to other bones or to nearby organs. On You-Tube I watch a video of one Robert Gallner from the United States explaining how he survived stage IV renal-cell carcinoma. I note that his tumour is the same size as mine and that he was able to have his surgery at the Mayo Clinic three short weeks after his growth was picked up by an ultrasound. He describes how the cancer came back and how he was operated on again. And then again. Robert displays a toy Roman soldier whose sword is raised and tells us that each time he went in for surgery or treatments he took the centurion along and imagined him fighting off the cancer cells. Robert's son, Alex, made the video and posted it to YouTube in 2009. Is Robert still alive? He provides an email address and I am tempted to contact him. Then I decide not to. No response, or a sorry note from his son, would be unbearable just now.

Dr. Finelli had mentioned a clinical trial that PMH is running to discover whether Sutent acts positively on renal tumours prior to surgery. I have decided against taking part, but Marie wonders whether it wouldn't be worth my while to speak with the oncologist Dr. Jennifer Knox, who is organizing the trial. She reminds me that the more doctors we speak to, the more information we receive. Not all doctors perceive a case in the same light: an oncologist, for instance, may have a slightly different take on my situation than a surgeon.

Dr. Knox, a tall blonde with a direct but sensitive approach, sets me straight on one thing: I had thought that after my surgeries, I'd be put on Sutent to ward off any further spread of my cancer. Dr. Knox explains that after my kidney and rib are removed, I am, technically speaking, free of cancer and do not qualify for the drug. I am disappointed hearing this; I was hoping for some assistance in keeping the cancer at bay, but Dr. Knox informs us that it isn't clear that Sutent can be effective in preventing the recurrence of kidney cancer. She surmises that the tumour has been growing inside me for a good ten years, and I wonder aloud, half-jokingly, what I did wrong ten years ago to engender my disease. Dr. Knox looks me straight in the eyes and says, "Of course, you did nothing wrong"—a gentle but straightforward reminder not to blame myself for my illness. She adds: "There *is* something odd about the biology of your tumour. I mean it's *huge* and yet it's done no damage to the nearby organs. And the rib that's affected is on your right side, not on the left near the cancerous kidney. It is a bit of a puzzle."

Doctors X and Y, as well as Dr. Finelli and the radiologists who have read my scans are fairly certain that (a) the tumour is cancerous and (b) the disease has spread to my ninth posterior rib.

Dr. Knox's puzzlement provides a modicum of hope, though I am hesitant to hope.

As the poet said: *Hope? / Nope.*

But I can't stop myself.

I take the pill of hope.

It's a little pill, but enough to buoy me for the next few days.

Tuesday, May 18

Our garden is thriving. I call it "our" garden, but in truth it is Marie's. I am the drone, following her instructions to dig here, move there. I am clumsy, unknowledgeable. Past springs I've dug up what I thought were incipient weeds and which turned out to be costly perennials planted the previous year. Now I ask permission before I uproot or prune anything. My tendency is to cut back in order to give the plants more space, but Marie's tendency has been toward a lush, densely populated garden. So the hostas and ferns intermingle beside the purple and lavender Siberian irises, the boughs of the pink flowering cranberry tree stoop over our deck. Later, white astilbes will cluster like patches of snow against their dark-green leaves. Marie stands back and considers. Deft in her decisions, she plucks and pinches, working long hours, never admitting to tiredness or thirst.

8

The garden shouts "health, health" and I am hoping that by working away in the earth and greenery I will be invigorated. But my joy is short-circuited when I consider that some of these plants may outlive me, may be greeting the sun after my demise. I am heartened to see that Marie looks good—it has been six years since her diagnosis. She is a slim, beautiful woman, moving gracefully and deliberately, with broad-brimmed sun hat and gloves, among the plants.

The work this morning conjures memories of gardens we have visited, most recently Francis Cabot's Quatre Vents garden in the Charlevoix region of Quebec. The variegated vistas, the sculpted light call attention to gardening's status as impermanent architecture, an indulgence of nature. I try to live in this May's moment of colour and perfumed air, delighting in the sight of Marie in her element, resilient, focused.

In the evening I read Virginia Woolf's essay "On Being Ill." Woolf had extensive experience from a young age with both psychological and physical illness—today she would be characterized as manic-depressive, or bipolar. She suffered from fainting spells, severe headaches, a weak and erratic pulse. These symptoms often left her bedridden, not necessarily a bad thing for a writer of striking originality.

As Woolf sees it, the healthy are engaged in mindless conformism; they act "with the heroism of the ant or the bee ... Mrs. Jones catches her train. Mr. Smith mends his motor. The cows are driven home to be milked." The healthy are allowed no respite from dreary routine. They must keep up the "genial pretence" in order to maintain the effort "to communicate, to civilise, to share, to cultivate the desert ..." But once we are taken ill she maintains that "this make believe ceases." Lying in our sickbeds, "we cease to be soldiers in the army of the upright; we become deserters. They [the healthy] march to battle. We float with the sticks on the stream ... able, perhaps for the first time for years, to look around, to look up—to look, for example, at the sky."

And what a "shocking" sight it is, "this incessant ringing up and down of curtains of light and shade, this interminable experiment with gold shafts and blue shadows." And to think, Woolf exclaims, that this "has been going on all the time without our knowing it!"

Woolf's meditation on illness soon becomes a satire on the mechanical activities of the robust who are blind to beauty, insensitive to nuance, blocked off from life's mysteries. Their conformism is the greater sickness. Woolf's patients are unconventional refuseniks. They blurt out the truth. They love to waste time and fantasize. I wish I could be more of a refusenik. I would like to practise greater indifference and cease worrying about the outcome of my surgery; I would like to spend more time contemplating clouds and the flowers in the garden. It is not enough for me to experience Nature—I must write about it, produce a tangible outcome from the experience. I suspect the same was true for the industrious Virginia Woolf. She too was a goal-oriented keeper of lists. In our own ways we continue, from our sickbeds, "to cultivate the desert."

Woolf's essay first appeared in T.S. Eliot's journal *The Criterion* in 1926. The most oft-quoted segment is the beginning, in which the author wonders why "illness has not taken its place with love and battle and jealousy among the prime themes of literature." In 1977, Susan Sontag noted, "Cancer is a rare and still scandalous subject for poetry." She said the same of AIDS in her 1989 book, *AIDS and Its Metaphors*. Have our attitudes changed since then?

There have been some inroads. Three years after Sontag's AIDS book, the well-known Anglo-American poet Thom Gunn received attention by publishing his collection of well-crafted and graphic AIDS poems, *The Man with Night Sweats*. Then, in 1998, Donald Hall published *Without*, a book of candid poems regarding his wife, poet Jane Kenyon, and her death from cancer. These were breakthrough books that helped to make serious illness a more acceptable theme in literature. There have been a slew of pop memoirs on illness—so many, in fact, that a journalist dubbed the genre SickLit. But serious considerations of illness in poetry and in prose are few and far between.

Wednesday, May 19

This morning I have a dentist's appointment. Just a regular checkup and cleaning. I don't know what shape I will be in after the surgery, so best to take care of such affairs now. In the afternoon I will have the hair on my balding head cut close to the scalp. I want to look clean on the operating table.

I've been thinking about Virginia Woolf's essay and how it puts a positive spin on illness. Her sick person is solitary and the happier for it. There's no attempt to describe the terrible aloneness the diagnosed person feels. I find that my illness exacerbates my native feelings of alienation. For me those feelings began in a home where emotions in general had to be capped and opinions calibrated so as not to offend. Speaking the truth was verboten. When I did defy the rules of emotion and assert myself, my words were met with silence or anger.

You spend a lifetime attempting to free yourself from the self-negation you learned early in life—those feelings, your therapist tells you, that are now "internalized." These problematic feelings make dealing with a life-threatening disease more burdensome. Sometimes you fail to see help when it appears, or you are wary of reaching out for it; you fear that you will be met with the same resentments that confronted you at home. That was a long time ago, but the ghosts live on, feeding off of the mental dynamic you have constructed for yourself.

On the transit ride to the dentist's I contemplate the variety of faces in the subway car. So many different lives, so many unknown stories. Who knows what drama each of them is living out behind the calm exterior? This is our silent pact: not to burden one another with our pain, our dread. When the hygienist who will clean my teeth asks me if anything about my health has changed, I lie and say no. I do not want to endure the ensuing pregnant silence. I do not want to watch her making a notation on my dental record. I want to be thought of as the same old me, cancer-free.

We are such fragile creatures. Like everyone else, I play a back-and-forth game between the image I have of myself and my image in the eyes of others. Like most, I swing between pride and humiliation with degrees in between. The time I spend among others at work, in a store, or in this dental office, opens me to gestures and words that have the power to bolster me or bring me down. And so I have gathered about me a small circle of family and friends in which I can reaffirm my self-worth. Now that I think of myself as sick, I find the affirmation more necessary.

Sickness has me revisiting some of the lonelier moments of my past. When I was ten we moved north of Sheppard Avenue, to a suburb under development. Urban pioneers, we were bombarded each weekday with the grunt of Caterpillar tractors, the echo of hammers, the whine of saws as the skeletal structures of houses sprung up around us. My mother found the place intolerable. The area was so new, it lacked bus service and she could not drive. Isolated, she withdrew, grew depressed, and took to bed for several weeks. I fixed my sister and me breakfast while our mother lay immobile in bed. When does literature enter one's life as a saviour? It was a few years after our move that I first read Shakespeare's *Hamlet*. It's astonishing how sensitive you become to language once you feel estranged:

> *Bernardo:* Who's there?
> *Francisco:* Nay, answer me: stand, and unfold yourself.

"Unfold yourself." Tell the truth. Reveal your identity. The first innocuous words of the play spoken by a night watchman resonated for me with extra intent.

> *Bernardo:* 'Tis now struck twelve; get thee to bed, Francisco.
> *Francisco:* For this relief much thanks: 'Tis bitter cold, / And I am sick at heart.

8

I, too, was sick at heart. Once you have identified strongly with a work of literature, reading can take over your life. I loved *Hamlet* the play for its patriarchal ghost and existential gloom. I loved Hamlet the character for his brooding and for his poetic speech. A few weeks after reading the play I watched Laurence Olivier's film adaptation of *Hamlet* on our Zenith television set. It's still my favourite film version of the play: the severe black-and-white cinematography; the atonal music, the sombre voice of Olivier played over the hypnotic surf of the northern sea.

Before my *Hamlet* encounter, my reading consisted of Hardy Boy mysteries and Tom Swift adventure books. From those I graduated to Ian Fleming's James Bond novels. It was my grade eight English teacher, Peter Wood, who introduced me to poetry. Wood, an amateur actor and singer as well as a lover of poetry, read aloud Emily Dickinson's "Because I could not stop for death— / He kindly stopped for me," and I felt—as Ms. Dickinson predicted I would—"as if the top of my head were taken off." The images and cadences of Dickinson's poem stuck in my mind, and as I walked home from school that frigid winter day, my own lines of poetry began to form in my mind. I was oblivious to my surroundings, completely absorbed in memorizing each line as it came to me. When I got home I rushed upstairs to my bedroom and jotted down the lines of my first poem. The following day I stopped at a bookstore on my way home from school and for fifty cents bought a paperback edition of Louis Untermeyer's *A Concise Treasury of Great Poems*. The first poem I read in that book was Keats's "Ode to a Nightingale." The poem struck a deep chord in me then, and now—forty-five years later and stricken with a potentially lethal disease—it speaks to me anew. Like the poem's narrator, I also long to escape, to fade away with the nightingale and "quite forget ... / The weariness, the fever, and the fret / Here where men sit and hear each other groan."

As a young teen, poetry became a life-sustaining passion, but it also exacerbated my alienation. No one in my immediate world read or wrote poetry. The activity was suspect for two reasons: first, it was impractical (i.e., not remunerative); second, it was considered unmanly. The culture I found myself in was dedicated to sports. It considered the athlete to be masculine, decisive, outwardly directed, while the artist was considered effeminate, uncertain, inward, and dreamy. As a young teen, I didn't have the courage to be an outsider. I was fortunate in that I was good at sports: I played hockey and baseball in our school's intramural leagues. I conscientiously hid my interest in poetry so that no one would think of me as an artsy geek. I recall surreptitiously scouring the shelves of the literature section during library period and heading back to my classroom with *The Poems of Robert Frost* sandwiched between a collection of grisly photos from D-Day and

a biography of baseball great Willie Mays, lest my male class-
mates see the Frost book and call me a "faggot," the term they
applied to readers of poetry.

8

After a few years in the suburban wasteland, our family moved
south to an established area and into an older house that my
parents had enlarged and renovated. This move provided
some happiness for my mother, as she was now within walking distance of shops. She busied herself with house improve-
ment, hiring an interior decorator and a German cabinet-
maker. My feelings of loneliness intensified as I attempted to
spread my adolescent wings, but my independence was met
with more hostility on the part of my parents. I was fortunate
in having a high school friend by the name of Herb Abrams.
Herb belonged to Mensa, owned some Lenny Bruce LPs, and
introduced me to the songs of Tom Lehrer. Herb's home environment was more sophisticated, due perhaps to the fact that
his maternal grandparents had been leftist intellectuals: his
mother was an amateur watercolourist and a serious reader
who kept Joyce's *Ulysses* on her night table. Herb's father ran a
successful optical business, but the family eschewed fancy cars
and clothes. One day on the walk home from school, Herb
handed me a Penguin paperback of Albert Camus's *L'Étranger*
(*The Stranger*). I can still recall the first words of the book:
"Mother died today. At least I think it was today ..." When I
got to the end, where Merseault stoically faces the cold blade
of the guillotine and Camus speaks of the "benign indifference of the universe," I felt as if my inner world had shifted
several degrees. After that it was Sartre's *Nausea*, *The Short
Stories of Ernest Hemingway*, Cyril Connolly's *The Unquiet
Grave*. Increasingly, my small book-lined bedroom became
my sanctuary amid a dysfunctional family. There I read and
jotted down quotations that impressed me. I wrote poems and
taught myself to play the guitar.

Literature and music were a comfort, but the discomfiting feelings I possessed remained locked inside. Can years of repressed emotions lay the seeds for cancer? In 1977, the year that Sontag's *Illness as Metaphor* was published, another notable cancer book appeared that wallowed in the sort of self-remorse and punitive thinking Sontag's essay cautioned against. The book was *Mars*, a memoir by Fritz Zorn. Zorn (German for "wrath") was the pseudonym for Fritz Angst (German for "fear"). The author, a thirty-two-year-old Swiss teacher, had been raised in a materially successful and highly repressive middle-class home. He describes his family as sterile, hypocritical—obsessed with social acceptability and lacking in any sort of affection or honesty. Zorn considers his cancer a call to arms (hence the title, *Mars*—the God of War), a last-ditch effort to speak the truth and clear the air. By changing his name from Fear to Wrath he hoped to release the poisonous feelings that he believed had contributed to his cancer.

Zorn blames his sickness on his suffocating family, and at one point in his eloquent indictment he bluntly states: "Anybody who is a good boy all his life deserves to get cancer." Have I been too good a boy? For years I taught apathetic college students who took my English course for a required credit. Unfulfilling work, to say the least. I wrote on weekends and in the summer. What if I had taken greater risks and tried to write full-time? Was my timidity, my allegiance to middle-class comfort, carcinogenic?

Zorn believes that no one gets sick unless he already is sick, by which he means living an inauthentic life. Do I believe that I gave myself cancer, that I willed my sickness? I find it disconcerting that, like Zorn, I am of the astrological sign Cancer (Latin for crab). It is not a particularly elegant sign if you consider the pincers and jaws of crabs. Nor is it a fortunate sign, since it reminds us of the link between the crab and our most dreaded disease. (The link is traceable to the ancient Greek physician Hippocrates, who found that a malignant tumour below the skin resembled the shape of a crab dug into the sand.)

Zorn likens the non-assertive Cancer type to a hermit crab withdrawing into his secluded shell. He finds reality too difficult. He is angry but directs his aggression back on himself. Franz Kafka was also a Cancerian. (He and I share a birthday, July 3.) Kafka viewed his illness (tuberculosis) as a reflection of his flawed personality. In a letter to Felice, his fiancée, he wrote: "secretly, you know, I don't believe this illness to be tuberculosis, or at least not primarily tuberculosis, but my all-around bankruptcy."

Self-flagellation often comes with sickness. I remind myself that it is an irrational response. Pent-up emotion does not cause cancer. I know people more repressed than I who are cancer-free. On the other hand, the French poet Arthur Rimbaud, wildly promiscuous and violent (one could hardly call him repressed) died of cancer at thirty-seven.

Cancer in most instances is random. Still I empathize with Zorn's wish to invest his disease with meaning. How terrifying it must have been for a thirty-two-year-old to think of his death as a soundless drop into the void. By blaming his family, by castigating his social milieu, he was able to focus his anger, articulate his despair, and rally his spirit while his bodily strength dwindled. In giving himself a cause, he asserted his identity. That sort of assertion is essential because being sick is often a dehumanizing process. In the eyes of doctors you become "a case." In the eyes of friends you become "the person with stage-IV cancer." In your own mind you can begin to think of yourself as little more than a failed specimen.

8

In recent times it has become fashionable for thinkers of a certain stripe to politicize their cancers. In Audre Lorde's *The Cancer Journals*, the African-American author blames white, paternalistic America for her disease. In Eve Ensler's recently published cancer book, *In the Body of the World*, the author, best known for her play *The Vagina Monologues*, blames her disease on our hostile imperialist society that has made it difficult for us to connect to our own bodies and to Mother Earth.

I have never been an overtly political person. I cannot connect my cancer to any ill-intentioned power structure. The abuse I suffered at the hands of my parents, or my youthful confrontations with what we used to call "the establishment," do not, in my mind, add up to cancer. As I see it:

> In the grand casino of life I have drawn a bad hand.
> The game I am playing does not allow me to discard.
> I must play the low clubs and hearts, the middling
>   diamonds and spades, as they come.
> I tell my story.
> My story will get me to the end.

Thursday, May 20

My friend the novelist and drama coach David Rotenberg has come through his own bout of cancer and advises me to stay in shape. "Keep exercising and you'll recover more quickly from the surgery," he advises me. David rode his bike several kilometres each day before his operation. I decide to remain faithful to my regimen of running and moderate weight-lifting.

I haven't often broken down during my wait time, though the other day, as I was jogging through the neighbourhood, my iPod Shuffle chose to play James Taylor's haunting a cappella version of "That Lonesome Road" and I unexpectedly lost it. I was touched by the angelic harmonies, the lyrics of loss, and the sincere tone of regret. I was moved by the song's admonishment:

> Never mind feeling sorry for yourself
> It doesn't save you from your troubled mind

I leaned against a lamppost and buried my head in my elbow and sobbed. Despite the admonishment from sweet baby James and his backup singers, I *was* feeling sorry for myself. I was thinking of Aiden and Jacob, my twin grandsons. I was hoping to live long enough to teach them to play the guitar. I'd already bought them ukuleles and got them strumming in rhythm to "Old MacDonald Had a Farm" and to "Wooly Bully," which they knew from a Chipmunks movie.

The thought of not being around for the boys saddens me. It is like being offered a glimpse into the future. Then the curtain is abruptly closed.

Friday, May 21

Thoughts of surgery. When my mother was in her early forties she felt numbness in her lower lip and jaw. Her GP thought it might be Bell's palsy but wasn't sure. For six months she ran to doctors who were unable to offer a diagnosis. It was her dentist who recommended she see a neurologist. Dr. Ross Fleming, at Toronto Western Hospital, watched her walk, watched her eye movements, asked her to spread her hands and bring her index fingers together, then told her he suspected a brain tumour. It was a benign tumour, an acoustic neuroma. Typically these tumours are slow-growing, developing on the main nerve leading from the inner ear to the brain. In some cases tumours of this sort can be left alone and "watched." Imaging techniques in the early 1970s were unreliable and the actual size of the tumour was unknown, but the numbness was not a good sign. It was suspected that her neuroma was fast-growing and large.

The operation lasted twelve hours. The surgeons removed a large piece of the back of the skull, and when we met with Dr. Fleming after the surgery he said that the tumour was significantly larger than they'd thought. "The size of a grapefruit," was how Dr. Fleming put it. It is a description that has always stuck in my mind. The surgery had turned out to be longer and more complicated than anticipated and there was a chance that my mother wouldn't make it. Fleming asked for our home phone number, in case he had to get in touch with us during the night. He also informed us that it would be a long road to recovery: the part of the brain that controls balance and mobility had been affected, and though it was an area of the brain that could regenerate itself my mother would have to learn to walk all over again, like a toddler.

She made it through the night. In the weeks following, infections developed that required further procedures. She moved from the hospital to a convalescence home where she learned how to walk. She fully regained her balance, but complained for years about the missing bone at the back of her head. The muscles in the back of her head, because they'd been cut into and because she used them to turn her head, were tight, uncomfortable, an annoying reminder of what she'd been through. After a number of years she stopped complaining about the tightness: either the situation remedied itself or she got used to the sensation.

I'm not expecting that sort of horror show. They are removing a kidney, and fortunately I possess another. As for the rib: I have plenty to spare. I've never been under general anesthetic. Marie describes it as "time out of time." You go out and then you come to with no sense of hours having passed. In those lost hours they'll have opened me and moved aside my spleen and my intestines and whatever else is needed to get at my cancerous kidney. Then they will sew me up and turn me over, and Dr. Y will come in and try her best to find the ninth posterior rib. Not the eighth. Not the tenth. The ninth.

Dr. Y is on my mind today because I'm heading down to PMH for another abdominal CT scan. I need this like a hole in the head, but Dr. Y wants to know whether the rib lesion has changed in size or if other lesions are developing. What are the odds that this scan will look different from the one I had seven weeks ago? I'm concerned: the radiation and nuclear dye are not kidney-friendly and soon I'll be flying with only one. Also, Marie has been keeping me secluded: she doesn't want me to catch cold or flu now that we are close to the surgery date. She frets that my trip for the CT scan will put me among the infectious. I've been trying to remain calm, focused, but this unexpected and likely unnecessary hospital visit is added stress. I email Dr. Tony Finelli for his opinion, which is dumb of me. Do I really expect him to interfere with another surgeon's directive? Predictably, he emails to say he must defer to Dr. Y on the matter and advises me to think positively. "Surgery is soon," he writes, "let's go into it positive, it will be reassuring if rib is unchanged."

Now why didn't I think of looking at it that way?

Saturday, May 22

The other day, Marie visited her father's grave. John died at fifty-eight and I am presently fifty-nine. I didn't have the heart to accompany her, so I have no notion of what she and John discussed. I do remember the choice location of John's grave under a broad-branched maple, so it is cool in the summer and strewn with yellow and rust-coloured leaves in autumn. Each time Marie went in for her cancer surgeries she wrote a farewell letter to each of our children. Just in case. I wouldn't call her a sentimental person, though I do think she has more feeling for people than I do. I can distance myself more readily.

I haven't written farewell letters or left instructions. Statistically, the odds that I survive my surgery are excellent. Afterwards, I may be lucky and live several years before a spot shows up on another bone or in my brain or liver. Death is not imminent, but I can't say that the thought of death hasn't touched me. Thinking about mortality confers a certain grace on your hours. You grow detached and see things around you dispassionately, as if from the grave. This sort of contemplation proves relaxing, an intermittent respite from angst: if I can envisage my not being here, I can confirm my expendability. I'm off the hook.

When I'm not in death mode, regret takes over. Regret is a huge part of serious illness. I've been nasty, and stupid, and wasteful with my time and talents: I can run up quite a score-card against myself. On the other hand, I'm proud enough to think that a few of my poems and essays will live. A consolation prize for bad luck on the health front.

Sunday, May 23

Last Thursday was our anniversary, but Marie and I decided to wait until today to celebrate. We're driving to a downtown restaurant that serves a halibut dish Marie fancies. She's behind the wheel and I'm in the passenger seat. I've been told I won't be able to drive for several weeks after my operation so I'm getting used to being driven around in our old Matrix.

Toronto is calm on a Sunday, not comatose, as it was during the 1950s, but tranquil nonetheless. We pass the intersection of College and Bathurst. On the northwest corner stands a church that has been converted into a condo and two doors west, at 462 College Street, is Lilliput Hats, where milliner Karyn Gringras produces exquisite handmade hats for women and men. The building was once owned by my grandfather and housed his tailoring business: Sherman Custom Tailors. Until the age of four I lived in the tiny one-bedroom apartment above the shop. My father and his two brothers worked alongside my grandfather and I spent many hours in the store when I was a child. Its images and sounds comprise a significant portion of my mental landscape.

At the front of the store my grandfather and my father would greet and fit their customers. The back section, where as a young child I pedalled my blue tricycle, was a mini-factory where the cutters, tailors, and pressers worked. I recall the long cutting tables and underneath them the large cardboard cartons for the scraps of discarded cloth. I recall the long, winding measuring tapes and little boxes containing white tailor's chalk, Gillette razor blades, and pins. Large spools of white thread fed the black sewing machines. Garment patterns the colour of dried blood dangled from hooks like sides of beef. Most fascinating to me was the ancient press iron with its long movable arm. I thought of the iron part, sleek and triangular, as the head of a prehistoric pterodactyl whose picture I had seen in a children's book on dinosaurs. The arm of the press iron was the creature's long neck and inside the head were tiny blue tongues of flame.

In the front of the shop the cloth samples hung like drapery on the walls. If the prospective customer could not find what he was looking for there, he was shown a catalogue of samples or led into the back, where bolts of cloth stacked to the ceiling in wooden cribs were unfurled with a flourish. I loved the names of the cloth patterns: herringbone, sharkskin, houndstooth, pinstripe, salt and pepper, tartan. And the textures: tweed, hopsack, twill, worsted, serge. I recall cloth unrolled on a large cutting table and men bent over, haggling over the price.

There would be a barrage of arguments or jokes that went back and forth between the workers in a mixture of English and Yiddish, and when they stopped their banter I could hear the careful closing of shears, the ripping of thread, the hiss of the steam press and the Gatling-gun clatter of a sewing machine that made a mockery of its name—Singer.

My father loved cats and would keep a number of them in the back of the shop. They'd been given extraordinary names: *No-Neck, Shvartz Katz, Rabinovitz.* They would doze on the cutting tables or sit like sphinxes atop the wooden cribs. My father kept a lint brush nearby to remove any of their hairs that had adhered to the cloth. There always seemed to be a cat that had just given birth, and for as long as I can recall there

were two signs in the shop's front window: one was professionally made and promised CLOTH—HALF PRICE. The other was
a large piece of cardboard on which my father had printed in
black marker: FREE KITTENS—ASK INSIDE.

Wednesday, May 26

6:45 a.m. Game time.

Marie has dropped me off at the Elizabeth Street entrance
to the Toronto General Hospital and gone to park. I enter with
morning shift workers who carry their lunch and hospital garb
in small knapsacks. I've got my night bag with flip-flops, pyjamas, toothbrush, and razor. Symptomless, I find it surreal that
I am about to submit to two major surgeries. I wonder, for a
moment, what would happen if I left the hospital and went
home and waited? How long before the tumour would cause
pain or impede my vital organs? Now Marie has greeted me
and I do not get to carry my thoughts any further, as we are
walking toward the elevators and making our way up to the
pre-op room. There I change into a pale-blue hospital gown
and put thin disposable slippers on my feet. I'm wheeled into
a large room where a number of pre-surgery patients are lined
up on one side of the room facing another row on the other. My
children, Justine and Adam, are here along with my brother,
Randy, who's flown in from Tampa to be by my side. It's good
to have familiar faces peering down at you, uttering words of
encouragement, before you go under the knife. Tony Finelli
is here too, dressed in his scrubs. He stops by and I introduce
him to my brother and my kids. He explains to me that before
the operation I will undergo a minimally invasive procedure
known as a renal-artery embolization in order to stop the flow
of blood to my cancerous kidney. Blood loss is an issue during
a nephrectomy (kidney removal) and surplus blood has been
ordered in case a transfusion is required.

An orderly wheels me into a room where two nurses and
two doctors are in attendance. Actually, one is a full doctor,

the other an intern. The nurses run an intravenous line into my arm and I'm given a sedative; the doctors pass a guide-wire and catheter into my right groin and are tracking its movement on the computer screen above my head. Embolization is from the Latin *embolismus*, to insert. I'm not sure what material they've inserted to plug the blood vessel, but I am surprised at how quickly this is accomplished. Everyone seems happy with the results they see on the screen. The doctor pulls the wire from my groin and wipes off the blood while I think of a dipstick drawn from an engine. Then the intern uses a cloth to press down on the insertion point to stanch the flow of blood. The bleeding won't stop and the intern is going through one drenched cloth after another. It occurs to me that I may require that transfusion Dr. Finelli has ordered even before I reach the operating room. Too bad the doctor's no longer here: he left the room the moment the embolization proved successful. "I'll let you finish up," he advised his intern, and sauntered out.

After a minute or two of frantic pressing, I suggest to the intern that he call the doc back to lend a hand.

"There's no way, that's not gonna happen," he barks at me, and continues with the desperate shoves to the groin.

When I first make the suggestion to call back the doc, the nurses flash me a peeved look (can't have a patient calling the shots), but several more blood-soaked rags and they too get jittery. I advise them that if this is going to go on much longer I'll need a top-up on the sedative and they comply. At least I'll be good and high by the time Finelli and Dr. Y get their hands on me.

It's amazing how detached a patient can become in such a situation. I am staring at the beads of perspiration that have formed on the intern's forehead. He's stressed and his breathing is more and more audible. His eyes—above his surgical mask and below his surgical cap—glare with worry, but eventually he gets the job done. I lift my gown and see that he's left a huge hematoma, an aching purple-and-rose bruise that extends down my inner thigh. The twit is walking out of the room without offering an apology, leaving behind a mound of blood-soaked rags for the nurses to clean up. I'm sedated, but the primal part of me wants to unplug the intravenous and go after him.

"Calm down," I tell myself. "You've got a long day ahead."

They wheel me back into the big pre-surgery waiting room. Most of the other patients have been wheeled off to their surgeries. I tell Marie what happened. She finds Finelli, who takes one look at my groin, winces, and says he's going to find a vascular surgeon to attend my operation in case there's an issue. I'm uplifted, watching Finelli speed down the hallway: the concerned physician, looking out for his patient. It's a good image to hold onto as I'm brought into the operating room, where two young anesthesiologists roll me onto my side to administer the epidural. They put a mask over my face and ask me to count, but I don't get far.

8

When I come to in the recovery room I am surprised by the intense pain. I wonder if the epidural failed to kick in. I tell the attending nurse that my back, the site of the rib surgery, hurts. She says this was anticipated and that they were waiting for me to awake before starting a morphine pump. The pump's a contraption that allows you to adjust the amount of morphine administered to your body so that you can manage your own pain. Later, the young anesthesiologist who attended my operation will visit my hospital room and tell me that the epidural hadn't been perfectly positioned. He wanted it low enough to cover the pain from the nephrectomy and high enough to counter the rib surgery. But the numbness didn't reach high enough to remedy the hurt of cut bone. He is very sweet and apologetic, and prescribes painkillers in addition to the pump. I'm someone who'd hated taking aspirin, but now I gobble down whatever pills I'm offered.

I think of myself as having a high pain threshold. I've had dental work done without any freezing; I can suffer through headaches until they dissipate on their own. The worst pain I can recall was when I had a severe case of the measles. I must have been eight or nine. I broke out in a raging rash on my face, chest, arms and legs. Light felt like a knife shoved into my eyes, and a fever-induced skull-splitting headache lasted days.

But this surgery is teaching me there is another dimension to pain. Each time I inhale, I feel a sharp, mean stab in my back where the rib was cut. They are working now at setting up the morphine pump. David Rotenberg told me the morphine caused him scary hallucinations; after a day on the pump he asked to be taken off. But at this very moment I'm anxious for them to start the drip. I need something to alleviate the stabbing sensation.

8

I am in my hospital room. It's a large room at the end of the hall and I am the only occupant. I have an intravenous line coming in and a catheter going out to carry my urine into a pail under the bed. I wear an oxygen mask and I have a plastic chest tube to drain off any excess fluid from the thoracic surgery. My left lower flank is heavily bandaged, as is my right upper back. Faces float by: my parents, my brother, my children. Marie is here, a constant. Other than the back pain, I'm feeling better than I anticipated. I doze off and then awake, relieved at the thought that the surgery is over. My window faces south on University Avenue and as the daylight wanes, the streetlights flare up. It is amazing to think that people, untouched by illness, are rushing along the street below. Even on the ninth floor I can hear, through the hermetically sealed windows, the faint hum of traffic. Those healthy walkers and bike riders and car drivers, rushing who knows where, are oblivious to their good fortune. They take time for granted. I'd like to join them in the land of the healthy, where death and illness are only fleeting apprehensions. Tonight, a few blocks north of here, at the Miles Nadal Centre, the Jewish community is handing out literary awards; my essay collection *What the Furies Bring* is being honoured. My father will read a brief acceptance speech on my behalf. My son, Adam, who has flown in from New York, has decided to stay with me tonight. There is a chair in this room that reclines into a makeshift bed, and he will sleep there to keep an eye on me. I tell him that it's not necessary, but he insists. When Marie had her cancer surgeries, Justine, our daughter, was away at Queen's University, writing exams for law school. Adam was a student at Western University in London. The surgeries took place over the Christmas break and he came in and helped me care for Marie. We'd go shopping together for carrots, onions, celery, and parsnip, and buy one large chicken cut into eighths. Marie had shown me how to make her unique, light-bodied chicken soup before she went in for her operations. The secret is to skim off a good deal of the fat. Adam and I learned to make a decent version of it in the weeks we were together. We were propelled by our love for Marie and by the joy of cooking together. When it was time for him to return to Western for the start of his second semester, he balked. He told me he wanted to stay and help out, but I told him that I could manage on my own and insisted he return. I recall standing with him at the Elizabeth Street station. We gave each other hugs and then he carried his overstuffed knapsack up the steps of the purring bus. It was a cold night and as I walked back to my car I looked up at the icy stars. Camus deemed the universe indifferent, but here on earth one finds love and compassion.

Thursday, May 27

The day after my surgery is the worst. I'm not doing too badly at 5:30 a.m., when Tony Finelli shows up to tell me that the surgery took much less time than expected and there was minimal blood loss. "The blood bucket under the operating table was nearly empty," he says. I appreciate the graphic imagery and tell him I'm feeling okay except for the rib pain.

In a few hours my pain increases significantly. The epidural is wearing off, so the site of the kidney incision is now hurting. The morphine pump has only a moderating effect on the rib pain and I begin to feel a stabbing ache in my upper chest that is intense and new. Coincidentally, as the pain mounts I receive my first visit from the pain-management team. In one of his stories Hemingway tells us not to trust doctors who travel in groups. These are doctors, Hemingway believes, who lack confidence in their judgments and skills. Heading the team is a young woman who holds a clipboard and asks me to rate my pain on a scale from 1 to 10. Describe the type of pain you are experiencing, she suggests. And then she scribbles. She checks the list of medications and says there is nothing else they can recommend for now. But they will visit again later. As the morning wears on, the upper-chest pain increases; at first the nurses and interns are stymied as to the cause. At around noon, my afternoon nurse comes on and wonders if the chest tube is causing the pain. This makes sense to me and I ask her to adjust the tube, but neither she nor the interns on the floor are allowed to touch it. The tube is the responsibility of the thoracic department and a call is put in for them to come and take a look. The next few hours are bad. It is as if an ice pick is poking into my chest each time I breathe.

It takes four excruciating hours for Dr. Y's intern to show up. Bulky, slow-moving, he checks the bandage covering my rib incision and tells me, in a thick Russian accent, that it is fine. He unwinds the tape holding the chest tube, pulls the tube out a fraction and—presto—the pain diminishes. "Try it like this," he says. Under other circumstances I'd be tempted to say, "Fuck you. What the hell took you so long?" but I'm so grateful that the pain has diminished that I feel like weeping and would gladly kiss his hand. Besides, I may need him to come back and readjust the tube.

They are measuring the amount of urine flowing into the container under my bed, monitoring the activity of my remaining kidney, which at first is hyperactive as it adjusts to its role as the single filter for the 200 litres of blood it must process daily. After several hours it settles down and performs as required. I will have to take extra good care of my kidney, since statistics show that losing one to cancer makes the surviving kidney more susceptible to disease.

I am being given a strong pain medication to augment the morphine. The morphine hasn't adversely affected me yet, other than to induce drowsiness. Under morphine, voices are minutely amplified, movements slowed a fraction, and the visual field discernably blurred through a whitish lens, as if everything were taking place under an angel's wing. But in the evening, Morpheus goes through a mood shift and appalling images drift by: gruesome shrunken heads, their eyes and mouths stitched shut, followed by the mutilated faces of decapitated pirates that stare at me and grin. My own private horror show. The faces dissolve into darkness then slowly reappear, accompanied by silver-eyed lizards and chattering monkeys.

At first I am perturbed, frightened, by the shrunken heads and scarred faces, but eventually I grow detached, inquisitive. It's like watching a film. Why these particular images? I ask myself. Why not erotic dreams or serene visions of suns setting over tropical islands? Are the frightful images fuelled by my apprehension of illness and death? Or are they visions common to patients under the influence of opiates? Late in the night they recede and I think of Thomas De Quincey's *Confessions of an English Opium Eater*, a book that gave weight and depth to my generation's all-too-common drug experience. The spectre of death hangs over the *Confessions*. I recall a passage where De Quincey describes an opium-induced dream in which he is a fleeing paranoiac buried with mummies and chased by disease-ridden crocodiles.

Friday, May 28

5 a.m. Today is better than yesterday. I'm off the hallucino-genic morphine pump and onto OxyContin. The pain has less-ened, I'm more alert, and I've just met my new nurse, Máire. "It's the Gaelic equivalent of Mary and pronounced the same," she informs me as she carefully draws the letters in felt pen on the whiteboard by the door of my room.

Máire is one of those nurses who can look you in the eye and convince you that it is your destiny to survive. She has what pop literature calls a "healing personality," which is a way of saying that she offers you her skill *and* her soul. Upon arrival she cleans house, establishes order, not because she has dictatorial impulses but because she cares. She checks my oxygen intake and tells me I no longer need my mask. She has me breathe into the incentive spirometer to upgrade my lung capacity. She removes my catheter and hands me a plastic pitcher for urinating. She informs me that I am going to go for a walk down the corridor—my first post-surgery walk—but that prior to that momentous event she will help me to the bathroom where I will disrobe and wash. With Máire I feel no shame. She helps me into fresh pyjamas and we begin our trek down the corridor. She elicits from me the feeling that I am her only patient: a helpful illusion as I begin my recovery.

She lets me know that I will not be permitted to leave the hospital until I have passed gas and urges me to let her know as soon as I do. I assure her that I will inform her the moment it happens. On second thought, I tell her, I'll wait a few minutes before calling her into the room. She smiles.

Adam has stayed with me for two nights and tells me he'll stay a third. I tell him that staying another night is unneces-sary, that I'm doing much better. We go back and forth on this. When Adam steps out of the room to get himself some break-fast, Máire, who has overheard our conversation, advises me to let him stay. "Did it ever occur to you," she asks me in a gentle voice, "that he wants to stay as much for himself as for you?" Actually, it hadn't occurred to me. I hadn't considered that staying would be a comfort to *him*.

At night, I have trouble sleeping and push my IV stand down to the nurses' station and talk with Rosie, a large woman from Jamaica. She tells me her concerns about the rough neighborhood in which she is singly raising her three kids, the gangs, the drugs, the chaos that reigns in the halls of the neighbourhood school. A little window into a life fraught with turmoil and worry. And there's Sarah, the lithe and handsome East Indian nurse who smiles broadly as she pads catlike down the corridor to help a patient.

The stories I heard beforehand, of patients calling for nurse at night and getting no response, are blasphemous. While Máire is exceptional, all my nurses are solicitous. Once at night, when I'd fallen asleep, I sensed a presence nearby and awoke to see Sarah shining a flashlight from the hall to check on me. My days in the urological ward have me thinking of nurses as the archangels of the medical system. I watch them at the nurses' station as they coordinate and co-operate effortlessly—a corps of super-female proficiency. (I've met no male nurses during my current stay.) I see them as a sorority of the caring, unspoiled by status, glamour, or power.

Saturday, May 29

You keep odd hours after surgery: you doze off during the day when you should be awake and lie awake at night contemplating your mortality. You're busy dealing with pain and discomfort and when they momentarily subside the brutal fact of your impaired biology intrudes and biblical truths strike home: ashes to ashes, dust to dust. You require a palliative to help you with the hard facts. During the day I read J.M Coetzee's essay collection *Inner Workings*, which my friend David Penhale has dropped off to speed my recovery. Here are elegantly written and insightful essays on Saul Bellow, Samuel Beckett, V.S. Naipaul, Italo Svevo, and the Roths (Joseph and Philip). I feel at home reading Coetzee's observations about works with which I'm familiar. But at some point in the night I tire of the written word and feel the need of a singer's voice to settle me.

I insert the earbuds of my iPod. The best cure for what ails me is the blues, and the best sort of blues proves to be the most elemental: Robert Wilkins's 1929 recording of "That's No Way to Get Along," Tommy McClennan's 1939 "Bottle It Up and Go," and Bill "Jazz" Gillum's 1940 version of "Key to the Highway." I love Ray Charles, B.B. King, John Mayall, and Eric Clapton, but in my present state (bandaged and hurting) I find their sound too produced. I'm searching for a raw voice with bare accompaniment: a keening harp, an upright piano, an acoustic guitar—something on which the naked soul can dance. I play a selection by Big Bill Broonzy or Blind Boy Fuller and I imagine a pool hall, a whorehouse, or a dingy tavern and a black man seated on a straight-backed chair, sliding the neck of a beer bottle over the strings of his beat-up guitar. His gravelly voice punctuates the room. He's Mr. Orpheus, just returned from a trip to the netherworld. A bottle of whisky— his payment for the evening—stands next to his stomping foot.

Why the blues? What other music bears witness to the individual's hard time? What other music approximates the poetry of solitude?

> They treated me like my poor heart
> was made of a rock or stone.
> You know that was enough, mama,
> to make your son wished he's dead and gone.

The music is not fussy, but the voice is loaded, complex. The singer can go from sexy to forlorn, from caustic to reflective, all in the same song. There is trouble in love and there is loving that is carried out in vain.

8

> Ain't it lonesome
> Sleeping by yourself

When the woman that you love
Is loving someone else?

There are train stations where your lady leaves you and crossroads where you meet the devil and highways where you roam until the break of dawn. Now that I am relegated to this hospital bed, now that I am a prisoner of my disease, songs of travel intrigue me.

The songs do not shy away from reality, and though they are not overtly political, they do recognize the meanness of the prevailing power structure:

Now, the nigger and the white man
Playin' set 'em up.
Nigger beat the white man
Was scared to pick it up

You have to hear Tommy McClennan's sardonic laugh after he finishes that verse to get the full impact. McClennan, born in 1905 in Durant, Mississippi, eventually moved to Chicago to play with other blues artists like Elmore James and Little Walter, and died there in abject poverty in 1962. Fellow blues musicians called him "Sugar." It is remarkable how the pain in his voice resonates with the emotional pain that I feel. Art transcending the specifics of time, place, and ethnicity, so that the travails of a black man from the South help heal the soul of a white man from the North who is recovering from cancer surgery.

My IV bag has run out and big-hearted Rosie has heard the warning beep. She smiles down at me as she deftly changes the bag and adjusts my pillows. I cannot lie on my left side due to the pain from the kidney incision; I cannot lie on my right because of the cut rib. I am restricted to lying in an upright position on my back and staring out through the darkened window at the lights running south through the streets of the city where people are searching for love and making their way toward the blues.

Sunday, May 30

Each morning two young technicians come into my room with a portable X-ray machine and take pictures of my chest. Today I ask them why and am told that after thoracic surgery there is a chance that the lungs might collapse. Their response has given me something new to worry about, but it is low on my list of concerns.

Shortly after the X-ray technicians exit, my pain-management team enters and asks me to once again rank my pain. I've grown impatient with this ritual and would like to respond sarcastically. I know they have nothing left in their arsenal to be of help. My body and soul are stretched out and I want to preserve my strength for the struggle ahead, but social convention persists and I grope for a digit that reflects my ride over rough terrain. "Four," I tell them, thinking I might just as well have said "three" or "five." The leader of the pack seems content with this and scribbles on her clipboard.

The same man cleans my room each morning. His ID tag tells me that he is Mohammed. I feel a connection to Mohammed, even though we don't speak much. I'm groggy in the morning, not up for conversation, but Mohammed and I smile at each other, a silent communication between two underdogs, hard-working immigrant and immobilized patient. The administration is justifiably terrified of C. difficile, the killing superbug, so Mohammed carefully cleans the windowsills, chairs, sinks, and mirror. He mops the floor each day, including the area under my high-tech bed.

There is something inherently vile about hospitals: the food is revolting, the noise is persistent, and no matter how much cleaning gets done there lingers a sense of filth: pus, phlegm, feces, urine, syringes, and bags of blood. The patient in the next room is ill and the staff is busy, trying to figure out whether his puking and diarrhea are related to his surgery or to a bug he's picked up. I'm hoping that it's not something contagious. I have enough to contend with.

Marie visits each day. I can picture the visitors' waiting room she sat in as I was operated on, awaiting news from Dr. Finelli—I sat in the same room during one of her surgeries. It is a spacious atrium, with comfortable couches and chairs that overlook the lobby of Toronto General. Intermittently, a doctor appears in cap and scrubs bearing news. One entire family takes a deep communal breath. Someone exclaims, "Thank God," and they all fall back, relieved. Another family sits tense, accepts the blow with bowed heads. Not long after Finelli came in with a thumbs-up and announced to my family that the operation was over, Marie went for a coffee and ran into Dr. Y in the corridor. Dr. Y told Marie she was relieved that she'd got the right bit of rib. Marie was glad about that too and said that maybe we'd be lucky and the rib tumour would prove to be benign. Dr. Y lowered her eyes and told Marie not to count on it.

I'm wearing a pair of blue-and-white pinstriped pyjamas, one of two pair that Marie bought for me before the operation. Previously, I was a man who did not own a single pair of pyjamas, preferring to sleep in a T-shirt. I also possess a newly purchased turquoise housecoat that I wrap about my hunched body each time I shuffle with my rolling IV stand down the corridor. Marie is meticulous about wardrobe and had bought the clothes I'd need for the hospital: oversized boxer underpants and a pair of summer shorts with an adjustable waistband to wear in the weeks after surgery, anticipating the swelling from the incision. I took this buying of clothes to mean I have a future. Who bothers to buy clothes for the dying?

Sometimes when I doze off, I find myself thinking of Marie rather than of my predicament. The nineteenth century French author Alphonse Daudet—who wasted away from advanced syphilis before the eyes of his wife and children— was overheard to say, "Suffering is nothing; it's all a matter of preventing those you love from suffering." Marie puts on a happy face for her daily visit, but I know she is sick at heart. She is plagued with over-responsibility at the best of times and

I know she is running a checklist of items involved in caring for me once I get home. I worry about her worrying. I would like to protect her from the suffering that comes from witnessing; I'd like to carry on with my notions of gallantry, but whom would I be fooling? When you've known someone for a long time, the shared suffering inevitably adds up.

I've tried my best to accept my role as patient. It's not a role of complete dejection. I swallow my palmful of pills; I take frequent walks, and wash regularly, even though it hurts to manoeuvre in and out of the tub. In truth, there's a certain status to being bedridden and there's a vacation aspect to the hospital stay. Domestic demands are on hold: no bill payments, no lawn-mowing, no house repairs. Out of sight, out of mind. I have to go back to childhood to think of a time when I've felt so completely unburdened. This is the angelic side of disease, the side that affords time to explore and probe; you take stock and pledge reformation, settle scores with yourself, and forgive others. You come to see everything around you dispassionately, as if from the grave. A great calm settles upon you; there are moments when you feel balanced, natural, like a stone or a tree.

The OxyContin supports your serenity. It's got its downside: fatigue, dizziness, itchy skin. I can't believe some people rob and kill for this stuff. And it constipates, when what you need is your bowels to start to churn so that the nurses know you're ready to leave.

Shitting: the subtext of many a patient's life.

When we were toddlers our first words of encouragement came as we were lifted off the potty.

As adults, we're grouchy until we have a good dump.

How much anxiety is attached to elimination? The great jazz musician Louis Armstrong was a firm believer in laxatives. He'd hand them out to friends and fellow musicians. He even offered a package to the Queen of England. He once posed for a risqué ad for the herbal laxative Swiss Krissly: the photo showed Satch on the toilet while the copy underneath read: Leave It All Behind, the "It" being not just your stool but also your troubles.

My stomach grumbles and I grow hopeful, expectant but nothing ensues. I know that my innards were pushed around during the surgery and that general anesthesia is itself constipating. There's a lot for my digestive system to work through. The Buddhists believe that if you obsess about a thing, it won't happen, so I try to keep my mind elsewhere and then, in true Buddhist form, I pass gas while walking through the halls of the ward. It is just a wee bit, but enough for Máire to congratulate me and sign off on my release.

Late in the afternoon a team of interns visits. Four serious heads. The leader of the pack sits down at the foot of my bed and asks how I'm doing. He tells me that they're thinking of releasing me tomorrow morning. He knows that I'm still in considerable pain, that I still need assistance. He asks if I have someone at home to help care for me. The one great problem in staying, he informs me, is that "something bad can happen." Those are his exact words and the bluntness surprises me. Patients believe they are hurried out of the hospital to free up beds, when in fact they are released because their odds of survival diminish with each additional hour they stay. A few minutes after the interns leave, my dinner is brought in. It's been nearly four days since I've eaten. Máire is standing by and says she hopes it's not the spicy-beef-and-noodles dish. "Some boiled veggies would be nice," she remarks as she lifts the tin lid. She groans. What sits on the plate resembles Purina Dog Chow that's been heated up and spilled over broad noodles. "God, they're stupid," Máire says.

8

Even the most philistine cancer patient becomes a brooding philosopher once he realizes that his time is brutally finite. The usual denials of mortality hold no sway for those diagnosed with metastatic cancer.

When I contemplate my death-nearness I feel a pang. I grope for an image to express the sense that life may be shortened. What was once a far horizon is now a distressingly close opposite shore, where dense woods abut the darkened waters. A rowboat is waiting for me. I am fairly certain that the woods I will walk through are eerily silent.

In this hospital setting there are long stretches of time and few diversions so my brooding can get out of hand. I awake from intermittent sleep without my glasses on and try to decipher the numerals on the schoolroom clock hanging on the wall opposite my bed. Time drips slowly, like my IV. My body needs these tubes and monitors and pills, but my spirit needs a respite from the facts. I count the minutes and groan.

I expected to have wild dreams after surgery, but sleep, when it has come, has been a blank slate. I have plenty to cope with while awake, so when I do zonk out my mind seems to shut down, recharging for the heavy psychological work ahead. But during my last night at Toronto General, I do dream.

A Dream of Leaving the Toronto General

I arise from my hospital bed
dress, walk out of my room
and down the corridor

the nurses do not recognize me
how can that be I wonder
I know I am the colour of a cadaver

In the elevator I stare straight ahead
avoiding the eyes of the orderlies

I walk into the street
and join the press of people
going their determined ways

It is a comfort to have a direction
my illness had made me desultory,

I have been riding death's wave
and now I once again am like
everyone,
like everyone I stride with the swell
of human traffic
anxious over things
that need doing

I reach the corner
and fix eyes with a street singer
I know no one in life has eyes
that intense that focused
his mouth moves soundless
he strums silence on his guitar
his plush-lined case
swings open like a coffin
and for a moment I panic
believing I've been walking
through the land
of the living dead

I toss him a coin and keep walking
blending with the crowd
hoping that he cannot see
the mark upon me.

Am I the character in my dream or is it my doppelgänger
(double-walker) who strides along the busy street? My dream
seems ominous, reminding me that my "I" may be the "fetch,"
a double figure who comes to fetch a man to bring him to his
death, or the Scottish wraith, an apparition seen by a person
just before death.

I have not resolved my feeling of having been marked.
Perhaps this writing is my way of dealing with the "why me?"
syndrome. I have been seeing my therapist once a week since
my diagnosis. He has *not* told me to think positively. He has
not assured me that things will be okay. From the very start he

was willing to accept the notion I put forward that this may not end well. He has allowed me to contemplate my death as a possibility, and that has been good medicine. The power of therapy rests on the idea that the recognition of one's reality and the reality of one's life are life-giving. Seeing my double in a dream is not necessarily a presentiment of death. In certain cultures, seeing one's double is synonymous with having attained some truth, and with the power of prophesy. There is the Talmudic legend of a man who, in search of God, meets himself. Would such a man go on to be a poet? A storyteller?

I have worked to get myself an earlier date for my operation. I have kept myself in shape so that my recovery would go more smoothly. And all the while I have kept an eye on the grave. I feel more authentic since my diagnosis, more grounded. My priorities have come into focus. I castigate myself for acting the fool for much of my life, for wasting valuable time, for wavering from the goal.

What was the goal?

To protect those closest to me and to work.

To tell the story.

Monday, May 31

Máire is off today. The nurse who takes her place pales in comparison. I was fortunate to have had a committed nurse to coach me during the first days of my recovery. I would not have progressed as quickly with another. And I am fortunate to be going home to Marie, who will pay attention to all the details of my recuperation, though I feel badly that she will have to care for me. Will this be too much for her? Is it true that everyone, after a time, tires of being a caregiver, no matter how loving and devoted?

Outside the hospital, the light has a perceptible density and for a moment I blink and flinch. I note pale patients in wheelchairs or in casts hovering around the semicircular drive, soaking up sunshine. The traffic noise, which I generally find

jarring, invigorates. I think of the Russian poet Varlam Shalamov who'd been exiled for close to two decades to the remot-
est edge of Siberia, where he was surrounded by a terrifying
silence. When he returned to Moscow he kept the window of
his downtown apartment open day and night through all sorts
of weather, claiming that the constant clang of the streetcars
gave him joy.

My brother and Marie pick me up around noon and we
drive north on Avenue Road, battling Toronto's heavy weekday
traffic. There's a shimmering quality to Avenue Road, with its
tony shops, its sunstruck elms and maples. We pass the offices
of dental surgeons and psychiatrists; we whizz by a health-
food emporium and a dealership specializing in exotic cars
for the stratospherically rich. In Toronto you can get the buzz
of urban living without the rash violence and desperation. It's
cautiously progressive, civilized—too civilized, according to
some. It proves to be a pleasant enough place to live in so long
as you can keep up a moderate pace and not fall too far behind
the pack. Marie and I have managed to hold on to our modest
two-storey house and my spirit lifts as we pull into the drive-
way. This has been my refuge for close to thirty years and I
know that my odds of recuperating here are good.

We've had rain and the hydrangeas in our front garden
have grown to a decent height. I can see buds forming. In
another month their white, confetti-like flowers will stand out
strikingly against the backdrop of dark-green leaves. The deli-
cately fringed Japanese maple, maroon in colour, bows slightly.
The boxwoods, yews, and emerald cedars thrive. Strange that
the sight of these flourishing plants makes me think suddenly of the diseased tumours that have been lifted from my
body. They were carried down to the basement lab at PMH
the day of my surgery. The kidney tumour was preserved in a
fixative and then sliced neatly into sections that were stained
and placed under a microscope. And not just the tumour. The
adrenal gland, the lymph nodes, the fatty tissue surrounding
the growth, the bone lesion that Dr. Y sliced from my ninth

posterior rib—all are being minutely inspected and written up in a dry and detached manner that in no way reflects the gnawing anxiety I feel at times, as I await word on whether or not death is pending. I have been advised that I will see Dr. Finelli on July 6 to find out the results of the pathology report. That is five weeks from tomorrow. If I had more strength I would have asked the nurse who handed me the appointment form as I was leaving Toronto General why I have to wait five weeks. It seems like an outrageously long time. But I am tired of fighting the System and, besides, I am fairly certain that the appointment will be a confirmation of what the docs have already surmised, with some encouraging words from Finelli thrown in about a wait-and-see approach and a schedule for follow-up scans and tests.

Sunday, June 6

I'm happy to be home, though I know I am now open to the dynamics of home life: arguments, the anxiety over malfunctioning garage doors, clogged toilets, the work of keeping the place in order. My pre-surgery fitness routine has indeed made the work of recovery go relatively smoothly. I begin to get back in shape by taking short walks around the block. I gradually build to longer walks that extend into distant reaches of my neighbourhood. My world, which a few days back was a hospital bed, and then a hospital corridor, is steadily increasing in scope.

The pain from the excised rib has subsided while the hurt from the kidney incision seems to have grown more acute. It's a raw burning sensation that penetrates from the inside out and has me stooping when I walk. The drug Percocet helps alleviate the pain but clogs my innards. The stool softeners and laxatives have done little to counteract the constipation, but the bottom line is that I am strengthening, in noticeable increments.

Yesterday we had a deluge of rain and at 6 p.m. the power went out. The blackout continued into the night. Marie and I read by flashlight. It's astonishing how quiet the world becomes when the electricity is off. I thought, This is the quiet that Shakespeare and Keats knew, the quiet behind the poems of Emily Dickinson and the intimate interiors of Vermeer. This is the quietude that existed before the world was hooked up to hydro poles. Marie has fallen asleep. I listen to her steady breathing and then I get up and walk to the bedroom window. The glass is beaded with humidity this warm June night. I peer out onto our street. The pitch-black houses across the road resemble hulks moored in a fog. No lamplight, no moonlight, no stars visible in the cloud-covered sky. A perfect stillness. In the dark and quiet I can envisage my annihilation. I began to assimilate the thought of dying shortly after I was diagnosed. I slowly realized that a person could imagine himself dead long before the body turns senseless. The blood circulates, but you have, psychologically speaking, prepared yourself for the end. As I peer out my window into the dark I think of our inability to integrate dying into the process of living and wonder if it is in part electricity, with its blaring lights and incessant hum, that impedes that assimilation. We are all online, we are all interconnected, and now it takes an act of will to separate from the deluge of information and chatter. It requires a conscious effort to stand and hear one's breath, to follow one's inner thoughts and be mindful that all things must pass.

Tuesday, June 8

Marie drives us north for a day to visit friends in the Haliburton region. I have always felt a deep connection to the lakes and rivers of northern Ontario. I spent my boyhood summers on them, fishing and canoeing. Now they mean something more:

Northern Lake

They've given you a name –
Ox-Tongue, Loon Call,
Big Bass, Turtle –

but long before names
you reflected shattered
sun,
mute clouds,
unconscious eye
of moon.

When the turbulence of wind
pushed you to the limit
you encased yourself in ice
and went silent.

What's nameless in me
goes with you.

You change,
you remain changeless
and these words are nothing more
than a way of making what vanished
permanent

as you lap away at rock
and nourish the deepening cold.

Monday, June 14

I have developed a painful lump on the underside of my middle toe and am heading down to PMH to have it checked out. My first anguished thought is that another cancerous bone lesion has formed, but the intern assures me that the lump is a tiny cyst that will likely disappear with time. The visit would have been forgettable had Marie and I not witnessed a heart-breaking scene in the waiting room.

A male orderly had wheeled a patient into the clinic and stood, along with the patient's distraught wife, before the glassed-in receptionist. I recognized the young receptionist from a previous appointment, when she'd taken forever to give me the schedule for a follow-up appointment. I politely questioned her about it and she snarled. The patient, a man in his seventies, was sick, slumped over in his chair, and obviously in no condition to respond when the receptionist informed him that he couldn't be seen by any of the doctors because, though he had his Ontario Health card with him, he did not have his Hospital Network card. The orderly spoke up for him, informing the receptionist that she was incorrect:

"He's an in-patient. He doesn't need a hospital card."

The receptionist dug in her heels. No card, no admittance.

"Look," the orderly said, raising the man's left arm to display his hospital wristband with full ID.

The receptionist shook her head no, at which point the patient's wife, a woman in her early seventies, obviously flustered and stretched beyond her limit, said, "I'm sorry. I must have forgotten the card in his room. I'll run up and get it."

The orderly offered to run up, but the woman preferred he stay and look after her ill husband. The wife returned empty-handed.

"I can't find it," she told the receptionist, gasping for breath. "I searched everywhere." She began to weep. And no matter what the orderly said to comfort her she couldn't stop weeping. She was an overweight woman and she wept convulsively, with her entire body. This, in front of a packed waiting room of fifty people. I felt a strong urge to throttle the receptionist. I was close by and saw the orderly glare at her and I knew that if any throttling would be done it would be he who would do it. She too noticed his glare and in response lowered her head and said, "All right, but next time bring the card." An apology, of course, was beyond her moral reach.

Are the cogs and functionaries who work at PMH given sensitivity training? As you sit in these crowded waiting rooms, or as you wait in line for your overdue surgery, you can't help but ask what is being done with the millions upon millions of dollars raised by Princess Margaret Hospital through its lotteries, its fundraising walks and bike rides, its full-page newspaper ads that present the personal testimonies of smiling survivors requesting donations? Is it all going into research, carried out far from the public eye? How much money goes to the CEOs of our mega-hospitals and to the heads of their fundraising foundations? I certainly couldn't see any influx of dollars as I joined the long queues for my tests and appointments.

Friday, June 18

Marie has filled three large pots with pink and white impatiens and sweet-potato vines. Each morning, before our walk through the neighbourhood, I water the impatiens with our garden hose. I write in the morning and read on the back deck in the afternoon, glancing now and then at the impatiens petals wavering in the breeze. After dinner, Marie and I talk on the deck. As the light wanes, the flowers grow more vivid. They glow in the dusk, asserting their beauty before the impending dark.

The pain from my surgery has abated and last night was the first time in close to a month that I was able to turn on my side in bed. I slept soundly until 3 a.m., when I was awakened by a familiar squeaking sound from above. It's difficult to tell if the raccoons have gotten into our attic or are foraging on the roof. Sometimes I hear them scratching in the eavestrough and know they are digging grubs and bugs out from under the dried leaves. Raccoon, from the Algonquian *arakhunem*, "he who scratches with the hands." They prowl through our neighbourhood, nervy, unabashed. Last week, I heard one rummaging in the garbage bin I'd left out for collection and went with a flashlight to scare it off. It looked up—the dark agates of its bandit eyes burning—then continued scaveng-ing, unconcerned by my presence. I returned to bed and lay awake, knowing that in the deep shadows a guerrilla pack of them were sniffing and snorting, uprooting plants and bulbs, plunging deep into trash. A reminder that nature is out there, waiting to take possession.

Tuesday, June 22

I wasn't aware, since I'd never before been operated on, that I am allergic to surgical tape. The skin around my kidney inci-sion has become raw and swollen. The terrible itchiness is a real concern and I've driven to my GP's office to see if a salve can be applied to bring relief. Sid advises leaving it to clear up on its own. He remarks on how good I look, and I tell him that I am feeling okay. In fact, I am feeling much better than I had anticipated four weeks after surgery. But my feeling of health is qualified.

There's a balance most of us maintain between our subjec-tive sense of self and the objective state of our bodies. Weight gain, hair loss, aging, disfigurement: our subjective self must adjust to the changes. (We know how difficult it is to adjust when we consider the money made in publishing diet books and in offering plastic surgery.) My physical disruption is internal, invisible, more complex. To look at me you would think I am the same person you always knew. The scars from my incisions are hidden by my clothes and will fade in time. But the cancer cells that likely remain within my bloodstream indicate that my time here may well be limited. I think of myself as housing a time bomb, only I don't know what the timer has been set for.

Tuesday, July 6

I am at PMH with Marie, waiting to hear from Dr. Finelli what the pathology report has to say. It is four months since Sid felt the swelling in my abdomen. Early on, my doctor friend Shel Krakofsky told me that what I'd been given were educated guesses and that until tissue is examined under a microscope, nothing is certain. I appreciated his attempt to provide a shred of hope.

The waiting room is less packed today; no doubt people are off on summer vacation, taking a respite from their jobs and cares. Each summer Marie and I spend a few days canoeing in Algonquin Park. If we don't make it north, we feel our summer is incomplete and that something essential has been denied. Both of us spent some of our youth in the northern part of the province, where the wild forests and lakes get under your skin and form a part of your identity. Last summer, paddling on Little Joe Lake in the early-morning light, we saw a moose with her calf come down and drink from the water; we saw them again the following morning on our return trip and took it as a lucky sign, though it hasn't been a lucky year for us.

Dr. Finelli is wearing his white lab coat (no purple shirt today) and greets us with an enthusiastic handshake. We sit down and he hands us a copy of the pathology report.

"It's good news," he says, flipping through the report. As it turns out, the tumour on my rib is benign. It takes a moment or two for this to sink in. I am happy and at the same disoriented: I have, after all, been living for four months with the thought that I have metastatic cancer.

I ask Finelli what sort of tumour I had on my rib.

"It's a xanthoma," he replies.

"What's a xanthoma?" I ask.

"Don't worry what it is." Finelli responds. "It's a good thing. Just take it."

I will, but I find Finelli's response to my question evasive. I want to know what fooled him, Dr. X, Dr. Y, and several of the radiologists at PMH so that they were compelled to open my back and remove a portion of my rib. Later, I will search the Internet and discover the following: "Xanthomas of the rib are extremely rare benign neoplasms, most commonly reported in soft tissue, but rarely in bone."

There is more good news. The kidney tumour is, as was expected, cancerous but confined to the kidney. No lymph nodes are involved. The tumour itself has been graded as a stage II rather than a stage I, since it is greater than seven centimetres in size. But cancer cells don't appear to be floating through my bloodstream, looking for another organ to invade. My cancer's histologic type is chromophobe. Ninety per cent of renal-cell carcinomas are of the clear-cell variety. Less than 5 per cent are chromophobe; one's chances of long-term survival seem to be slightly better with the chromophobe variety. There is one minor hitch: Finelli has found a discrepancy in the report; the pathologist claims that the cancer has invaded the surrounding fatty tissue, which would make the tumour a stage III rather than II.

"It doesn't make much difference," he explains. "The survival odds for a stage II are 85 per cent, for a stage III, 75 per cent. The important thing is that we're not dealing with metastatic cancer. That is a completely different disease." He will ask for clarification from the pathologist, whom I note by glancing down at the report, is Dr. Joan M. Sweet. The following day Dr. Sweet will amend the report in my favour: there appears to be no invasion of the fatty tissue.

I am pleased, though I am not jumping up and down. After all, I have had a fifteen-centimetre cancerous growth cut out of my body along with my kidney and part of a rib. But I am relieved, very relieved, to know that my situation is not as dire as I had imagined and that I may live into old age.

Am I triumphant? It's a common reaction when one has recovered from a life-threatening illness. Many patients savour it; some even grow boastful. I admit to a sense of triumph, but I resist it: it's bad form to act as though you are out of the woods when in fact there are still several kilometres to go. I recently read on the Internet the testimony of a doctor whose stage II kidney cancer returned fifteen long years after he was initially diagnosed. So what is there to crow about? Furthermore, "triumph" implies that I fought a battle. I didn't; I merely got a lucky break. Nothing I did or thought caused my cancer, or caused it to be less than what the doctors surmised; nothing I do or think will keep it at bay. I try my best not to take responsibility for the cause or progress of my illness, only for its psychological and spiritual ramifications.

Finelli informs me that during the first year I will have an ultrasound every three months. After that it will be an ultrasound every six months, along with an abdominal CT scan. These will be periods of "scanxiety," the term psychologists give to those times when, no matter how fine a patient feels, the fear of a malignant spot showing up will overtake him and he will live in dread until he receives reassurance that all is clear.

Thursday, July 22

We're at PMH again, this time for a follow-up with Dr. Y. "Don't count on it," was what she had said to Marie when Marie suggested that the bone tumour might not be malignant. Now Dr. Y is blushing and apologizing for what turned out to be a needless surgery. I bear no grudge: I tell Dr. Y not to worry, and express hope that in the future imaging techniques will advance to where a lesion can be identified as cancerous or not *prior* to surgery. She examines my back; there is a prominent indent where the piece of rib was removed; when I breathe, the skin moves in and out like the bellows of an accordion. I ask Dr. Y if flesh and muscle will ever grow to fill the gap and she shakes her head no.

Monday, March 7

It is close to a year since I was diagnosed and in that time I have written several book reviews, three longish essays, and a number of poems toward a new collection. I have resigned from my teaching position at the college. How would I feel if my cancer returned and I was doing a job I no longer loved? The only work that makes me feel completely whole is this work of shaping language.

Kidney Cancer Canada is hosting a presentation by Dr. Andrew Matthew, a psychologist at PMH, titled "From Patient to Survivor." I don't care for the term "survivor" when it comes to cancer. I think of the doctor whose early-stage kidney cancer lay in wait for fifteen years and then crept up on him and said, "Boo!"

I prefer to think of myself as a post-operative cancer patient.

According to Dr. Matthew, up until 2004 the psychosocial care provided by hospitals to cancer patients was negligible. It is somewhat better now, he believes, thanks largely to the Lance Armstrong Foundation's push to acknowledge the emotional plight of cancer patients. But sadly, most hospitals still treat only the physical aspect of the disease. In study after study, cancer patients complain that their psychological needs are not being met. Dr. Matthew stresses the traumatic nature of hearing a diagnosis, the ensuing numbness, anger, denial, and the excruciating sense of isolation. He outlines the emotional repercussions facing patients after treatment including depression, fatigue, lethargy, and fear of recurrence.

In the question-and-answer period I ask Dr. Matthew what sensitivity training doctors are given. He repeats my question into the camera (his presentation is being broadcast online) and snickers, as if to say, "Are you kidding?" Then he regains his professionalism and tells us that doctors spend a very brief time in med school on how to deal with emotional situations. Then I ask Dr. Matthew if he has ever offered his presentation to the doctors at PMH, so that they too may gain insight into the emotional turmoil of the patients they treat. He has not offered his presentation to doctors. I am tempted to ask Dr. Matthew, a staff psychologist at PMH, why he has not offered his presentation to doctors at Canada's premier cancer centre. Does he fear he wouldn't get a supportive turnout?

It's a shame that physicians are not more attuned to these emotional issues. A doctor—especially a doctor dealing with terminally ill patients—may not know that he or she can be as much a victim of the System as the patient. Not every patient can be cured or saved, but his spirit can be eased by the way he is treated by his doctor. And in responding to the patient, the doctor may discover that he heals himself. Is it possible for the doctor to get beyond his distancing techniques and preserve his equilibrium? Would he, in fact, be strengthened if he drew his patient closer, if he saw his patient fully as a person rather than as a case? Is it possible for both the patient and the doctor to share the sickness experience, for them both to feel what it is like to be on the edge of existence? Or is this asking too much?

8

It is a year since my kidney and rib surgeries. The ultrasounds over the past twelve months have shown several miniscule lesions on my liver, which are too small to characterize. These have caused some worry, though Dr. Finelli is confident they are "nothing." My most recent ultrasound—two weeks ago— was carried out not by a technician but by a young intern in radiology. He was smart, upbeat, and expert at performing the ultrasound. He told me that this was my lucky day, and when I asked him why, he said, "Because today Dr. Kim is the radiologist who'll be reading your results. He is a world expert on liver imaging."

When I meet with Dr. Finelli, I find out that Dr. Kim has resolved the matter: the lesions are deemed to be harmless hemangioma. At the end of the brief meeting, Dr. Finelli looks me in the eye and tells me that he can never forget my case. I'm taken aback; he must have hundreds of cases to deal with. Why, I ask, does mine stand out?

"When you came to us we thought your situation was exceptionally grim and yet it turned out exceptionally well. It rarely goes that way."

He never let on that he thought my situation was "grim," which is just as well. I had enough negativity of my own to deal with.

It heartens me to know that my case means something to Dr. Finelli. I have given him a story in return for the excellent care he extended me, and stories, after all, are precious. They are a potent medicine against pain and suffering

Not only for the patient, but for the doctor, too.

8

If Marie or I should ever get sick again it would be good to continue our ritual of going to the Hope Street Café, but the restaurant closed six months after my surgery. Where will we ever find an eatery with such an evocative name?

At night we hold each other. Our illnesses have brought us closer together, with a deeper understanding of our temporality. When Marie lays her hands on my abdomen and massages me I know that she is wishing the cancer to stay away, and I suspect she senses the same when I touch her.

With time, our scars fade. Memory fades, too. My fear is that as the months and years pass I will become complacent and careless with Time. I will see Time as those who are blessed with health see it: an unending horizon.

I will forget what I learned when I looked back from the edge of life.

Acknowledgements

A segment of this book previously appeared in *Brick* magazine 95 (Summer 2015). The poems in *Wait Time* first appeared in the following journals: *Exile Literary Quarterly* ("Heart," "Umbrella," and "A Dream of Leaving Toronto General"), *Vallum* ("Northern Lake"), and *Stand* (UK) ("Venus Occluded").

I want to thank David Penhale and Ken Hundert for reading early versions of the manuscript, and Chandra Wohleber for her comments and encouragement. I owe a special thanks to Lisa Quinn and Robert Kohlmeier, who have proven to be resourceful and discerning editors. Of course, the book would not have been written without the support of my wife, Marie.

Notes

Part One

page v   "Sickness sensitizes man" Edmond and Jules de Goncourt, entry of 27 March 1865, in *Pages from the Goncourt Journal*, trans. Robert Baldick (New York: NYRB, 2006).

page v   "There is, let us confess it" Virginia Woolf, "On Being Ill," *The Moment and Other Essays* (London: Hogarth, 1947), 17.

page v   "The patient has to start" Anatole Broyard, *Intoxicated by My Illness* (New York: Fawcett, 1992), 20.

page xiii "The Angel of Disease" Kenneth Sherman, *What the Furies Bring* (Erin, ON: Porcupine's Quill, 2009).

page xiv   "scandalous subject" Susan Sontag, *Illness as Metaphor*, in *Illness as Metaphor / AIDS and Its Metaphors* (New York: Farrar, Straus and Giroux, 1990), 20.

page 19   "the radiant immediacy" Harold Brodkey, *This Wild Darkness: The Story of My Death* (New York: Holt, 1996), 110.

page 25   "Hope is slavery" Varlam Shalamov, *Kolyma Tales*, trans. John Glad (London: Penguin, 1994), 469.

page 29   "Thou hast brought me" King James Version, Psalm 22:15.

page 30   "The man suffering from a characterized sickness" E.M. Cioran, *A Short History of Decay*, trans. Richard Howard (New York: Arcade, 1975), 14.

page 39   "The conference's keynote speaker" Kidney Cancer Canada's conferences and meetings can be viewed online: http://www.kidneycancercanada.ca.

page 40   **"It's not death I fear"** Leonard Cohen's interview with Jian Gomeshi on YouTube: https://www.youtube.com/watch?v=ugh8Xe6hX7U.

page 43   **"the results can be miraculous"** These drugs are known in the pharmaceutical world as multi-kinase inhibitors. They not only stop angiogenesis but can dramatically slow the proliferation of cancer cells throughout the body.

page 43   **"nothing is extraneous"** Dr. Siddhartha Mukherjee, *The Emperor of All Maladies: A Biography of Cancer* (New York: Scribner, 2010), 388.

page 45   **"One must live"** "Interview with Boris Pasternak," *The Paris Review* 25 (1960).

page 45   **"Heinrich Heine's 'Schopfungslieder'"** Quoted in Walter Kauffmann, *Nietzsche: Philosopher, Psychologist and Antichrist* (Princeton, NJ: Princeton University Press, 1975), 130.

page 45   **"Poetry is a health"** Wallace Stevens, *Opus Posthumous* (New York: Knopf, 1957), 200.

page 45   **"Ernst Pawel's superb biography"** *The Poet Dying: Heinrich Heine's Last Years in Paris* (New York: Farrar, Straus and Giroux, 1995).

page 46   **"I am currently rereading Harold Brodkey"** Brodkey, *This Wild Darkness: The Story of My Death* (New York: Holt, 1996); Gillian Rose, *Love's Work* (New York: Schocken, 1997); Donald Hall, *Life Work* (Boston: Beacon Press, 1993).

page 46   **"Cast a cold eye"** Final lines of "Under Ben Bulben," in *W.B. Yeats Selected Poetry* (London: Macmillan, 1962).

page 51   **"there is a Midrash"** Martin Buber, "Kafka and Judaism," *Two Types of Faith* (London: Macmillan, 1951).

Part Two

page 59   **"Freud loved work"** For a discussion of Freud's work habits see Peter Gay's *Freud: A Life for Our Time* (New York: Norton, 1988).

page 59   **"When Freud grew old"** For an account of Freud's illness and death see Max Schur, *Freud: Living and Dying* (Madison: International Universities, 1972).

page 60   **"special dispositions and gifts"** Sigmund Freud, *Civilization and Its Discontents* (New York: Norton, 1962), 27.

page 61   **"I didn't think it would be useful"** Susan Sontag, *AIDS and Its Metaphors*, 101.

page 62   "deform the experience" Susan Sontag, *AIDS and Its Metaphors*, 102.

page 62   "the most truthful way" Susan Sontag, *Illness as Metaphor*, 3.

page 63   "random, spontaneous mutations" George Johnson, "Random Chance's Role in Cancer," *New York Times*, 19 January, 2015.

page 63   "the sick man sees everything" Broyard, 7.

page 63   "metaphors may be as necessary to illness" Broyard, 18.

page 63   "a small bird" Brodkey, 49.

page 63   "the truth of the Imagination" Keats, letter to Benjamin Bailey, 22 November 1817, in Walter Jackson Bates's *Keats* (New York: Oxford 1966).

page 63   "a parallel species" Mukherjee, 38.

page 64   "Cancer cells can grow" Mukherjee, 6.

page 64   "long after her treatments" David Rieff, *Swimming in a Sea of Death: A Son's Memoir* (New York: Simon and Schuster, 2008), 28.

page 65   "I'm responsible for my cancer" Rieff, 36.

page 65   "I feel like the Vietnam War" Rieff, 35.

page 65   "my mother's steely resolve" Rieff, 156.

page 67   "the term 'psychopoetics'" Ulrich Teucher, "The Therapeutic Psychopoetics of Cancer Metaphors: Challenges in Interdisciplinarity," *History of Intellectual Culture* 3, no. 1 (2003), http://www.ucalgary.ca/hic/files/hic/teucher.pdf.

page 68   "wait times for different types of surgeries" These can be found at http://www.waittimes.net.

page 75   "the sterility went too far" Broyard, 55–56.

page 80   "Hope? / Nope" Robert Zend, "The World's Shortest Pessimistic Poem," *The Maple Laugh Forever: An Anthology of Comic Canadian Poetry*, ed. Douglas Barbour and Stephen Scobie (Edmonton: Hurtig, 1981).

page 82   "the heroism of the ant or the bee" Woolf, 19.

page 82   "we cease to be soldiers" Woolf, 18.

page 82   "unconventional refuseniks" For an insightful discussion of Woolf's essay, see Hermione Lee, "Prone to Fancy," *The Guardian*, 18 December 2004.

page 82   "illness has not taken its place" Woolf, 14.

page 83   "graphic AIDS poems" Thom Gunn, *The Man with Night Sweats* (London: Faber and Faber, 1992).

page 83   "candid poems regarding his wife" Donald Hall, *Without* (Boston: Houghton Mifflin, 1998).

page 87   **"benign indifference of the universe"** Albert Camus, *The Stranger*, trans. Stuart Gilbert (London: Penguin, 1961).

page 88   **"Anybody who is a good boy"** Fritz Zorn, *Mars* (London: Picador, 1982), 220.

page 89   **"secretly, you know"** Kafka, letter to Felice Bauer of 30 September 1915, quoted in Ernst Pawel's *The Nightmare of Reason: A Life of Franz Kafka* (New York: Vintage, 1985), 382.

page 89   **"blames white, paternalistic America"** Audre Lorde, *The Cancer Journals* (San Francisco: Aunt Lute Books, 1997).

page 90   **"hostile imperialist society"** Eve Ensler, *In the Body of the World* (New York: Henry Holt, 2013).

page 102   **"an opium-induced dream"** See the "Pains of Opium" chapter in Thomas De Quincey's *Confessions of an English Opium Eater* (New York: Signet, 1966), 96.

page 108   **"Suffering is nothing"** See Julian Barnes's introduction in Alphonse Daudet, *In the Land of Pain*, trans. Barnes (New York: Knopf, 2002), x.

page 112   **"a double figure who comes"** The fetch, the wraith, and the Talmudic legend are discussed in the chapter "The Double," in Jorge Luis Borges's *The Book of Imaginary Beings*, trans. Norman Thomas di Giovanni (New York: Dutton, 1978).

page 114   **"kept the window of his downtown apartment open"** For a biography of Varlam Shalamov that includes this detail, see http://russiapedia.rt.com/prominent-russians/literature/varlam-shalamov/.

Books in the Life Writing Series
Published by Wilfrid Laurier University Press

Haven't Any News: Ruby's Letters from the Fifties edited by Edna Staebler with an Afterword by Marlene Kadar • 1995 / x + 165 pp. / ISBN 0-88920-248-6

"I Want to Join Your Club": Letters from Rural Children, 1900–1920 edited by Norah L. Lewis with a Preface by Neil Sutherland • 1996 / xii + 250 pp. (30 b&w photos) / ISBN 0-88920-260-5

And Peace Never Came by Elisabeth M. Raab with Historical Notes by Marlene Kadar • 1996 / x + 196 pp. (12 b&w photos, map) / ISBN 0-88920-281-8

Dear Editor and Friends: Letters from Rural Women of the North-West, 1900–1920 edited by Norah L. Lewis • 1998 / xvi + 166 pp. (20 b&w photos) / ISBN 0-88920-287-7

The Surprise of My Life: An Autobiography by Claire Drainie Taylor with a Foreword by Marlene Kadar • 1998 / xii + 268 pp. (8 colour photos and 92 b&w photos) / ISBN 0-88920-302-4

Memoirs from Away: A New Found Land Girlhood by Helen M. Buss / Margaret Clarke • 1998 / xvi + 153 pp. / ISBN 0-88920-350-4

The Life and Letters of Annie Leake Tuttle: Working for the Best by Marilyn Färdig Whiteley • 1999 / xviii + 150 pp. / ISBN 0-88920-330-x

Marian Engel's Notebooks: "Ah, mon cahier, écoute" edited by Christl Verduyn • 1999 / viii + 576 pp. / ISBN 0-88920-333-4 cloth / ISBN 0-88920-349-0 paper

Be Good Sweet Maid: The Trials of Dorothy Joudrie by Audrey Andrews • 1999 / vi + 276 pp. / ISBN 0-88920-334-2

Working in Women's Archives: Researching Women's Private Literature and Archival Documents edited by Helen M. Buss and Marlene Kadar • 2001 / vi + 120 pp. / ISBN 0-88920-341-5

Repossessing the World: Reading Memoirs by Contemporary Women by Helen M. Buss • 2002 / xxvi + 206 pp. / ISBN 0-88920-408-x cloth / ISBN 0-88920-410-1 paper

Chasing the Comet: A Scottish-Canadian Life by Patricia Koretchuk • 2002 / xx + 244 pp. / ISBN 0-88920-407-1

The Queen of Peace Room by Magie Dominic • 2002 / xii + 115 pp. / ISBN 0-88920-417-9

China Diary: The Life of Mary Austin Endicott by Shirley Jane Endicott • 2002 / xvi + 251 pp. / ISBN 0-88920-412-8

The Curtain: Witness and Memory in Wartime Holland by Henry G. Schogt • 2003 / xii + 132 pp. / ISBN 0-88920-396-2

Teaching Places by Audrey J. Whitson • 2003 / xiii + 178 pp. / ISBN 0-88920-425-x

Through the Hitler Line by Laurence F. Wilmot, M.C. • 2003 / xvi + 152 pp. / ISBN 0-88920-448-9

Where I Come From by Vijay Agnew • 2003 / xiv + 298 pp. / ISBN 0-88920-414-4

The Water Lily Pond by Han Z. Li • 2004 / x + 254 pp. / ISBN 0-88920-431-4

The Life Writings of Mary Baker McQuesten: Victorian Matriarch edited by Mary J. Anderson • 2004 / xxii + 338 pp. / ISBN 0-88920-437-3

Seven Eggs Today: The Diaries of Mary Armstrong, 1859 and 1869 edited by Jackson W. Armstrong • 2004 / xvi + 228 pp. / ISBN 0-88920-440-3

Love and War in London: A Woman's Diary 1939–1942 by Olivia Cockett; edited by Robert W. Malcolmson • 2005 / xvi + 208 pp. / ISBN 0-88920-458-6

Incorrigible by Velma Demerson • 2004 / vi + 178 pp. / ISBN 0-88920-444-6

Auto/biography in Canada: Critical Directions edited by Julie Rak • 2005 / viii + 264 pp. / ISBN 0-88920-478-0

Tracing the Autobiographical edited by Marlene Kadar, Linda Warley, Jeanne Perreault, and Susanna Egan • 2005 / viii + 280 pp. / ISBN 0-88920-476-4

Must Write: Edna Staebler's Diaries edited by Christl Verduyn • 2005 / viii + 304 pp. / ISBN 0-88920-481-0

Pursuing Giraffe: A 1950s Adventure by Anne Innis Dagg • 2006 / xvi + 284 pp. (photos, 2 maps) / 978-0-88920-463-8

Food That Really Schmecks by Edna Staebler • 2007 / xxiv + 334 pp. / ISBN 978-0-88920-521-5

163256: A Memoir of Resistance by Michael Englishman • 2007 / xvi + 112 pp. (14 b&w photos) / ISBN 978-1-55458-009-5

The Wartime Letters of Leslie and Cecil Frost, 1915–1919 edited by R.B. Fleming • 2007 / xxxvi + 384 pp. (49 b&w photos, 5 maps) / ISBN 978-1-55458-000-2

Johanna Krause Twice Persecuted: Surviving in Nazi Germany and Communist East Germany by Carolyn Gammon and Christiane Hemker • 2007 / x + 170 pp. (58 b&w photos, 2 maps) / ISBN 978-1-55458-006-4

Watermelon Syrup: A Novel by Annie Jacobsen with Jane Finlay-Young and Di Brandt • 2007 / x + 268 pp. / ISBN 978-1-55458-005-7

Broad Is the Way: Stories from Mayerthorpe by Margaret Norquay • 2008 / x + 106 pp. (6 b&w photos) / ISBN 978-1-55458-020-0

Becoming My Mother's Daughter: A Story of Survival and Renewal by Erika Gottlieb • 2008 / x + 178 pp. (36 b&w illus., 17 colour) / ISBN 978-1-55458-030-9

Leaving Fundamentalism: Personal Stories edited by G. Elijah Dann • 2008 / xii + 234 pp. / ISBN 978-1-55458-026-2

Bearing Witness: Living with Ovarian Cancer edited by Kathryn Carter and Lauri Elit • 2009 / viii + 94 pp. / ISBN 978-1-55458-055-2

Dead Woman Pickney: A Memoir of Childhood in Jamaica by Yvonne Shorter Brown • 2010 / viii + 202 pp. / ISBN 978-1-55458-189-4

I Have a Story to Tell You by Seemah C. Berson • 2010 / xx + 288 pp. (24 b&w photos) / ISBN 978-1-55458-219-8

We All Giggled: A Bourgeois Family Memoir by Thomas O. Hueglin • 2010 / xiv + 232 pp. (20 b&w photos) / ISBN 978-1-55458-262-4

Just a Larger Family: Letters of Marie Williamson from the Canadian Home Front, 1940–1944 edited by Mary F. Williamson and Tom Sharp • 2011 / xxiv + 378 pp. (16 b&w photos) / ISBN 978-1-55458-323-2

Burdens of Proof: Faith, Doubt, and Identity in Autobiography by Susanna Egan • 2011 / x + 200 pp. / ISBN 978-1-55458-333-1

Accident of Fate: A Personal Account 1938–1945 by Imre Rochlitz with Joseph Rochlitz • 2011 / xiv + 226 pp. (50 b&w photos, 5 maps) / ISBN 978-1-55458-267-9

The Green Sofa by Natascha Würzbach, translated by Raleigh Whitinger • 2012 / xiv + 240 pp. (5 b&w photos) / ISBN 978-1-55458-334-8

Unheard Of: Memoirs of a Canadian Composer by John Beckwith • 2012 / x + 393 pp. (74 illus., 8 musical examples) / ISBN 978-1-55458-358-4

Borrowed Tongues: Life Writing, Migration, and Translation by Eva C. Karpinski • 2012 / viii + 274 pp. / ISBN 978-1-55458-357-7

Basements and Attics, Closets and Cyberspace: Explorations in Canadian Women's Archives edited by Linda M. Morra and Jessica Schagerl • 2012 / x + 338 pp. / ISBN 978-1-55458-632-5

The Memory of Water by Allen Smutylo • 2013 / x + 262 pp. (65 colour illus.) / ISBN 978-1-55458-842-8

The Unwritten Diary of Israel Unger, Revised Edition by Carolyn Gammon and Israel Unger • 2013 / ix + 230 pp. (b&w illus.) / ISBN 978-1-77112-011-1

Boom! Manufacturing Memoir for the Popular Market by Julie Rak • 2013 / viii + 249 pp. (b&w illus.) / ISBN 978-1-55458-939-5

Motherlode: A Mosaic of Dutch Wartime Experience by Carolyne Van Der Meer • 2014 / xiv + 132 pp. (b&w illus.) / ISBN 978-1-77112-005-0

Not the Whole Story: Challenging the Single Mother Narrative edited by Lea Caragata and Judit Alcalde • 2014 / x + 222 pp. / ISBN 978-1-55458-624-0

Street Angel by Magie Dominc • 2014 / vii + 154 pp. / ISBN 978-1-77112-026-5

In the Unlikeliest of Places: How Nachman Libeskind Survived the Nazis, Gulags, and Soviet Communism by Annette Libeskind Berkovits • 2014 / xiv + 282 pp. (6 colour illus.) / ISBN 978-1-77112-066-1

Kinds of Winter: Four Solo Journeys by Dogteam in Canada's Northwest Territories by Dave Olesen • 2014 / xii + 256 pp. (illus.) / ISBN 978-1-77112-118-7

Working Memory: Women and Work in World War II edited by Marlene Kadar and Jeanne Perreault • 2015 / viii + 246 pp. (illus.) / ISBN 978-1-77112-035-7

Wait Time: A Memoir of Cancer by Kenneth Sherman • 2016 / xiv + 138 pp. / ISBN 978-1-77112-188-0

Also by Kenneth Sherman

Poems

Black River

The Well: New and Selected Poems

Clusters

Open to Currents

Jackson's Point

The Book of Salt

Relations: An Anthology of Family Poems

Black Flamingo

Words for Elephant Man

The Cost of Living

Snake Music

Prose

What the Furies Bring

Void and Voice: Essays on Literary and Historical Currents